Diabetes Recovery:

Reversing Diabetes
with the
New Hippocratic Diet™

Irving A. Cohen, M.D., M.P.H.

www.ForgetDiabetes.com

Center for Health Information
Topeka, Kansas
www.centerforhealthinformation.com

Published by
Center for Health Information, Inc.

1919 SW 10th Ave., Suite 22F
Topeka, KS 66604

Library of Congress Control Number: 2010902766

Cohen, Irving A. 1944-

Diabetes Recovery:
Reversing Diabetes with the
New Hippocratic Diet™

Includes Annotated Bibliography and Index

ISBN 978-0-9820111-0-2

Editor, Alice Heiserman
Cover Illustrator, Darlene Powell

Printed in the United States of America

This book is dedicated to those who are hoping to conquer type 2 diabetes.

Warnings and Disclaimers

- Diabetes is a serious and life-threatening condition. Therefore, decisions to alter therapy and/or diet should not be taken lightly and advice should be sought from a physician who understands the available treatment options.

- All readers are urged to obtain medical evaluation and support. Nothing in this book should be construed as individual medical advice. The reader should consult his or her own physician for such advice.

- Recipes and food choices discussed in this book are intended for those following this plan. These may or may not be the best choices for others.

- The information presented in this book has been obtained from sources believed to be authentic and reliable. Although great care has been taken to ensure the accuracy of the information presented, the author and the publisher cannot assume responsibility for the validity of all the materials or the consequences for their use.

Contents

Other Books by Dr. Cohen

Doctor Cohen's New Hippocratic Diet™ Guide: How to Really Lose Weight and Beat the Obesity Epidemic

Center for Health Information

ISBN 978-0-9820111-9-5

Cooking for the New Hippocratic Diet™

Center for Health Information

ISBN 978-0-9820111-7-1

(available soon)

Addiction: The High-Low Trap

Health Press

ISBN 0-929173-10-4

To check availability, or order these
or to order additional copies of this book,
go to

www.CenterForHealthInformation.com

Acknowledgements

In my earlier book of this series, I stated "There are so many people and circumstances that have influenced or helped me along the way to completing this book. Many may not have realized the contribution they made or the impact of their influence on me. This list will be incomplete, for I am sure that when I finish, others will come to mind." This is equally true for this book.

I will, once again, begin by thanking my patients. Many diabetics came to lose weight, both because they were unhappy being overweight, and because they had been told that their diabetes could be better controlled, once they had lost weight. Most were surprised at how rapidly their disease came under control, early in their weight loss. Their focus shifted to making continued control of diabetes their primary objective, with weight-control an added bonus. They had the courage to believe their test results, sometimes in the face of skepticism of others.

Again, I would like to acknowledge the pioneers who recognized both the cause of the obesity problem and the solution long ago. The works of Hippocrates and Wilhelm Ebstein regarding weight-loss demonstrate that there is little new under the sun. To that list, let me add the physicians of ancient India, who clearly saw the cause and effect relationship between dietary change and *Prameha,* which we recognize today as type 2 diabetes. Many doctors in the late nineteenth and early twentieth century were advocates of appropriate dietary therapy for diabetes, especially Arnaldo Cantani and again Wilhelm Ebstein.

However, it took physicians, chemists and engineers of recent decades to develop and perfect the diagnostic testing and instrumentation that have proved invaluable in providing diabetics the tools that make this approach practical. Using the monitoring now available strengthens the dietary approach developed so long ago.

Once again, I would like to thank the Sisters of Charity of Leavenworth, Kansas for reaching out to provide care for the uninsured through the Marian Clinic of Topeka and to Mary Stewart, ARNP for her help in working with these needy people. Special thanks go to those institutions that preserve and make available knowledge of past centuries, especially:

- Clendenning Library of the History of Medicine at the University of Kansas School of Medicine, Kansas City, Kansas (Dawn McInnis, Rare Book Librarian)
- National Library of Medicine, History of Medicine Department, Bethesda, Maryland
- Bibliothéque Interuniversitaire de Medécine, Histoire de la Medécine, Paris, France

Again, special thanks go to my editor, Alice Heiserman. Finally, my wife, Lauren, whose own family has felt the burden of diabetes, has stood by me in this mission to bring help to others. Thank you.

Introduction

This book is specifically for type 2 diabetics, their families, and friends. Two years ago, after my book *"Dr. Cohen's Guide to the New Hippocratic Diet: How to Really Lose Weight and Beat the Obesity Epidemic"* was published, I noticed a trend. People who had been referred to me by other physicians already had developed significant health problems. Since then, as the obesity and diabetes epidemics have continued to worsen, a greater percentage of the people referred to me are burdened with the dual problems of overweight and type 2 diabetes.

When this plan is carefully followed, they have not only lost considerable body weight but more importantly, achieved better control of their diabetes while reducing or eliminating their diabetic medication.

The diet guide included information for physicians and diabetics, for the extra attention needed in these situations. This book is expanded with additional information specifically to benefit those with type 2 diabetes.

Diabetics should use it with the supervision of their personal physician. Any significant dietary change will, by its nature, require careful monitoring of a diabetic who is taking medication. Done properly, this process can be highly effective and safe.

Irving A. Cohen, M.D.
Topeka, Kansas

<u>Warning</u>

You will not understand this plan by thumbing through, speed-reading, or skimming this book.

Some people who have tried many diets think they can understand any diet by quickly browsing and recognizing a word that they have seen in another diet.

As you read this book in its entirety, you will find that there are many principles considered here that have never been considered in other popular diets and plans. Recognizing a word here-and-there does not mean you understand what is about to be said, and you may skip reading what could be a very important chapter.

Please, do not start this plan unless you are willing to fully read this book.

Myths and Half-Truths

Do you believe in the tooth fairy or the Easter bunny? Probably not; yet, you may believe many of the myths and half-truths attempting to explain why you are both overweight and diabetic. Many of these myths are keeping you from successfully controlling your diabetes and losing weight. You are not to blame. Popular media and well–intentioned government agencies all have helped to spread misinformation. Pharmaceutical companies have a special interest in keeping it that way. Achieving better control of your type 2 diabetes while getting to a healthier weight will mean setting aside much of what you thought you knew. How many of these wrong ideas do you believe?

1. Diabetics always gets worse.
Half-truth!

Yes, type 2 diabetics often get worse, if their diabetes is poorly controlled. In that case, they may require ever more medication and develop serious complications. However, for many diabetics, major dietary changes can reverse the course of their disease. Better control of their blood sugar levels can then prevent further deterioration and sometimes allow healing of organs that were injured by high sugar. When better diabetic control is coupled with weight-loss, this can lead to major health improvements over time.

2. Diabetics <u>Should Not Try</u> for perfect glucose control.
Half-truth!

Doctors and scientists clearly understand that better control of blood glucose will result in less organ and blood vessel damage. The problem is that when this has been tried in large-scale experiments using diabetic medication, the medication forces blood sugar to go too low, resulting in major harm and even increased risk of death. This has resulted in physicians trying to adjust their patients´ medication to keep glucose levels under moderate control but avoiding attempting to get hemoglobin A1c levels into a normal range.

In other words, when using medication to control blood sugar, physicians no longer attempt to get you all the way back into a normal range. This minimizes the danger of overshooting the mark, but only slows down the progression of disease. However, by using diet alone, you may be able to safely bring your glucose level into a normal range. If you can do this successfully and continually, you can hold or even reverse the progress of disease.

3. It is the weight-loss that brings diabetics under better control.
Half-truth!

Both weight-loss and significant changes in diet each can

improve diabetic control. Taken together, weight-loss and sustained dietary changes support each other, resulting in significant improvements. However, of the two, I believe that dietary changes alone produce the greatest benefit. I say this, even though I am an advocate of weight-loss. Often, I see type 2 diabetics normalize their glucose levels and come off diabetic medication early in their weight-loss program, even before there have been dramatic changes in their weight.

4. Weight-Loss Diets Cannot Work
Myth!

Tell my patients that weight-loss can not work. They have lost extraordinary amounts of weight that they had been carrying around for years, despite their many unsuccessful weight-loss attempts in the past. This includes both those with significant disease and those who were still otherwise healthy. The most successful went on to have a lifestyle change. As these dieters became more aware of what had caused their past diet failures, their attitudes about themselves changed. A diet that works both effectively and naturally not only helps people lose weight and regain their health but also helps them to develop more positive feelings about themselves. For some, successful dieting gives them the confidence to now succeed in many other aspects of their lives, as well.

5. Overweight People Lack Willpower
Myth!

Do you believe that you lack willpower? Many overweight people have significant self-esteem issues because of this myth. Eating the wrong food actually changes your body chemistry. An ineffective diet can cause you to be constantly hungry when you are trying to lose weight. Your body is chemically signaling you to eat more and so, you do. You are not weak-willed. You are responding to a bad diet. You did not fail; the bad diet failed you.

6. Inherited Metabolism Keeps You Overweight and Causes Diabetes
Half-truth!

Yes, genetics plays a role in both overweight and type 2 diabetes, but less than people believe. True, some people may have a family with many people who are overweight and diabetic. Others may have a thyroid disorder, which slows metabolism, but this is easily identified through a simple blood test and corrected through thyroid medication. Both "slow metabolism" and "a genetic curse"are convenient ideas to hang on to when you think that you are doing the right things and yet still gain weight.

Two of the groups that have been most maligned about this supposed genetic curse are Native Americans and Americans of African ancestry. **Yet, historically both of these groups were once fit and slim. Genetically, they still carry that heritage to be fit and slim**. Economic conditions burdened them with unhealthy diets long before the remainder of our nation became obese. Today, people of all heritages are in the same boat. Even nations such as India and China are now experiencing epidemics of obesity and diabetes as they move toward our industrialized food ideas.

7. People are Fat Because They Do Not Exercise
Half-truth!

I heartily approve of reasonably increased exercise for any dieter. However, it is wrong to say that people would not be overweight if they exercised more. This is a gross oversimplification. Exercise will build muscle strength, improve body tone, and help your self-esteem. However the amount of exercise needed to accomplish any significant weight loss can be enormous. Exercise may aid both your weight-control and diabetic program, but it should never replace diet.

Have you ever been to a gym where an exercise group is being led by a twenty-something young lady in spandex? If you are fifty pounds overweight and find it impossible to follow the exercise routine she is leading, think about how much she would be able to accomplish if she had a fifty pound backpack strapped on! You are already exercising just by carrying around your extra weight. You are neither lazy nor incompetent because you are worn out by carrying this extra burden during your daily activities.

8. Certain Types of Food Will Burn Off Your Fat
Myth!

There are no magic answers nor are there magic foods! Diets that tell you to eat foods that match your hair color or similarly ridiculous ideas do not work. Everyone wants to believe that there are quick and easy answers. How many diet books do you have on your bookshelf that promised magic? The only way a weight-loss diet can work is by changing your metabolic balance so that you burn up your stored energy. The real magic is learning about the right mix and amount of food that allows you to eat less without feeling hungry or deprived.

9. Eating Fat Makes You Fat
Myth!

Eating more food than your body needs makes you fat, in whatever form it takes! Your body is programmed to take any extra energy you provide and store it for emergencies and lean times. Ounce for ounce, fat does contain more energy than any other food, but that fact is meaningless. To store fat, your body needs to receive a signal from insulin. In non-diabetics, a high sugar level drives that insulin level! In diabetics, the very medication you take may worsen your weight problem.

The quickest way to get fat is to stuff yourself with any form of carbohydrate that will turn into sugar. Farmers and ranchers have known this since ancient times. That is why cattle and poultry are fattened by feeding them grain.

10. Cholesterol is Bad for You.
Half-truth!

It is true that an imbalance of cholesterol is bad for you, but cholesterol is an important and vital necessity. Without cholesterol, your body could not make many hormones that are essential to life. The problem with cholesterol occurs when your body creates too much "bad" LDL cholesterol and too little "good" HDL cholesterol. Simply lowering your total cholesterol number without differentiating between good and bad cholesterol can do more harm than good. The right diet can help you achieve a healthy cholesterol balance.

11. Low-Fat Dieting is Effective and Healthy
Myth!

Several very large studies recently completed backfired on the proponents of low-fat dieting. In those studies, large groups of women were followed for an extended period of time. **The studies showed low-fat dieting to be _highly ineffective_ for weight loss.** In addition, low fat usually means increased proportions of carbohydrates. These high-carbohydrate diets can lower your good HDL cholesterol and worsen your diabetes.

12. Diabetics need carbohydrates.
Myth!

Diabetics who are not on medication do not need any minimum amount of carbohydrate in their diet. However, once started on diabetic medication, substantial amounts of carbohydrates are usually included in the recommended diet to prevent hypoglycemic reactions from the medication. *It is like your pet chasing its own tail.*

13. "Natural" sugars are healthier than refined sugars.
Myth!

All sugars are essentially the same. Your body will turn all of them into glucose, the sugar that is the universal currency for sugar-energy in your body. Some may be a little slower; some may contain impurities if less refined. These are expensive money-makers for the companies that sell them, but you can become just as diabetic from unrefined sugar or fruit sugar as you can from other forms.

14. All Natural Foods are Healthy
Half-truth!

Yes, **real** natural foods are usually healthier, but government regulators have responded to the food processing industry and distorted the meaning of the word "natural"on a food label. Because of this legal mislabeling, you may mistakenly be purchasing artificial "Frankenstein foods" thinking that they are healthy and natural. Instead, these unnatural foods can keep you addicted to overeating. Since not all "natural foods" are equal, you must become aware of foods that are causing diabetes and obesity.

15. A Fat-Burning State is Bad for You
Myth!

A fat-burning state is bad for a Type 1 diabetic when it is associated with high glucose levels. In that case, it is a marker for being dangerously out of control. This is not the case for others. The advice in this book is intended for type 2 diabetics. You **must** put your body into a fat-burning state to lose a substantial amount of fat. An ideal diet keeps your body burning the energy it stored as fat without destroying other tissues. Staying in this state reduces your blood sugar to normal levels and allows your system a chance to recover from the insulin resistance that the high sugar levels caused.

Nature has provided us with the ability to store large amounts of fat as energy to be used in lean seasons. In industrialized nations, most of us do not have large seasonal variations in our diet nor do we go into hibernation as animals do. Therefore, we may constantly overeat, without ever going in to a steady fat-burning state. This simply results in our just continuing to get bigger. When we store energy in the form of fat, we must switch over to a fat-burning state to get rid of it.

16. Surgery may be the Only Answer for a Heavy Diabetic
Myth!

A growing number of people have lost weight and achieved better control of diabetes as a result of surgery that radically altered their digestive tract. Why was this necessary? Should half of the industrialized world require surgery to be healthy? In addition to its high monetary cost, there is a significant physical cost. Surgery has its drawbacks and once done, you are never the same. The goal of surgery is to modify the amount and way you digest your food. Some people who have undergone surgery may learn to "eat around" their limitation and regain their lost weight, leading to tremendous disappointment and despair.

There is another answer. Instead of surgery, learn how a natural plan can reduce you appetite and allow your body to regain control of energy metabolism. A diet that works can save you from surgery.

17. Diet Drugs May Help
Half-truth!

Yes, some drugs can help you lose weight by eating less, burning more energy or interfering with food absorption. However, there is a high price to pay, with side-effects that may endanger your life. This is especially true if you already have high blood pressure or heart disease as a result of your diabetes. Recently, the European Union recommended that a diet drug popular in the United States be banned, due to excess deaths.

The pharmaceutical companies are spending billions of dollars in research to develop new diet drugs. Drugs that promise miracles generate blockbuster profits for drug companies.

Those who lose weight by using drugs do not learn how their body can naturally maintain weight and may have to continue on drugs for the rest of their lives to maintain their weight-loss.

18. Advice from Magazines and the Internet is Reliable
Myth

If advice from magazines and the internet were reliable, you probably would not be reading this book. Pharmaceutical companies, food companies, and soft-drink companies all have a vested interest and have spent hundreds of millions on public relations "spinning" the truth. Money influences research, even at major institutions. Trade groups front phony organizations, which are designed to look like they are consumer-run. Even legitimate professional organizations have given in to the lure of industry support. The profits from you being sick are enormous. The food-pharmaceutical complex is making billions as you become sicker. Be very skeptical. If you already know that the approaches they have recommended do not work, do not keep trying them. A quote attributed to Albert Einstein defines insanity as repeating the same ineffective action and expecting it to work the next time.

This book will teach you about a plan that has worked for many, both to lose weight and control diabetes. The New Hippocratic Diet™ is a starting point to begin this journey. As you progress, you will be learning about changes that will keep your diabetes under control as you lose weight. Read and understand this plan before you start. Obtain the cooperation and advice of your personal physician. Although no plan can be a perfect fit for everyone, many overweight diabetics have changed their lives using this plan.

Diabetes is a serious disease.
Do not start this plan unless you are prepared
to make the effort to follow it.

All you have to regain is
your health and your self-esteem.

2

What Is This Plan About?

- **What is the *New Hippocratic Diet,*™ *and how can it help diabetics*?**

This plan is based upon the *New Hippocratic Diet*™ which is a weight-reduction diet that emphasizes maintaining a steady state of fat-burning. I developed a computer model to predict the fat-burning potential of weight-reduction diets. That model showed that the key factors in maintaining efficient fat-burning are the following:

- Keeping a balance between the amount of food in your diet versus your total energy needs
- Keeping the proportions among fat, protein, and carbohydrate in your diet balanced for your weight-reduction needs.

This allowed me to develop techniques for producing a diet providing an effective method for weight-reduction. One group who needed this most were overweight people who had already developed type 2 diabetes. I have been selective in recommending this plan to diabetics, because it requires careful monitoring and cooperation of their other treating professionals, to prevent dangerous hypoglycemic episodes that would result from too much diabetes medication as their diet changed. As diabetics began to use this program, it became obvious that there was a tremendous benefit to them. They were able to both come off diabetic medication while achieving **better** control of their blood sugar levels than they had achieved on medication.

- **Why is fat-burning important?**

Keeping your body in a steady fat-burning state signals your brain that you are relying on burning stored energy. This state of a high degree of fat-burning reduces your appetite and minimizes your sugar-based food craving. This is important for diabetics.

Type 2 diabetes usually begins with insulin resistance. This occurs because bodies of type 2 diabetics are producing too much insulin in response to dietary intake of too many substances that will raise their blood sugar. Eventually, the cells that are designed to respond to insulin start doing this more reluctantly. At that point, blood sugar rises even higher and the cycle of type 2 diabetes has begun.

However, typically, the initial problem actually began earlier. Their bodies valiantly attempted to accommodate this high sugar intake, until they could not keep up any longer. By changing their metabolic state, they are less reliant on insulin to burn energy. This very change allows a rest for the insulin-resistant cells and may help them to return to more normal functioning. Some type 2 diabetics may also go on to develop insulin insufficiency. That means that they may be less capable of producing enough insulin for their needs. By emphasizing a fat-burning state, their actual insulin need may be greatly reduced, allowing for better control.

- **Why is this a *plan* and not just a *diet*?**

Type 2 diabetics can benefit tremendously from the New Hippocratic Diet™. Those benefits will come about long before reaching any weight-loss goal and will continue beyond that goal, provided that they are consistent in following this plan. Their need is greater than a weight-loss dieter without similar medical problems. Therefore, they should not consider this just another way to lose weight, but a plan to bring their disease under control.

- **Why is it *Hippocratic*?**

I used my computer model to predict an optimum diet for weight-reduction that differed from popular diet recommendations commonly seen today. Curious, I did historic research and I found two important historic diets that relied upon these same principles. One was developed by Wilhelm Ebstein, a respected German physician and scientist of the late nineteenth century. That diet was widely used and highly effective in its day and continued to be found in American medical texts well into the twentieth century. The other was the weight-reduction method of Hippocrates, the father of rational Western medicine. When I evaluated the Hippocratic principle of weight-reduction with my twenty-first century computer model, I realized that Hippocrates got it right.

Chapter 2   *What is this Plan About?*

- **Is this like other diets attributed to Hippocrates?**

No, for many years, the name of Hippocrates has been misused, to add credibility to useless ideas. When I look at popular diets and websites, it would appear that there are many statements and claims used for sales purposes. Fortunately, almost two centuries ago, a famous French scholar, Emile Litré, devoted a good part of his life to gathering, evaluating, translating, and producing the most complete and authoritative collection of Hippocratic works yet produced. My knowledge of what Hippocrates <u>actually</u> recommended is based upon the foundation provided by Litré.

- **Do other diets emphasize fat-burning?**

Yes, many of the carbohydrate-avoidance diets <u>attempt</u> to do this. Two of the most best known recent examples of carbohydrate restrictions were the diets of Dr. Robert Atkins, during the 1970s and again in the 1990s, as well as Dr. Irwin Stillman's in the 1960s. Both popularized low-carbohydrate diets that <u>intended</u> to reduce appetite by inducing the fat-burning state known as *ketosis.*

In actuality, neither was original. Both borrowed from earlier ideas and ignored some basic human physiology in attempting to produce a fat-burning state. These diets did work for many, simply because the foods available at that time matched some of the correct mixtures needed. However, as our food supply changed radically, following their ideas often results in poor results.

People who do not understand the physiology of dieting think this diet is similar. That is far from true. Although their diets recognized that high carbohydrate consumption cancelled out fat-burning, they misunderstood the interplay between fat and protein. By calling for too much protein, they ignored a basic issue, since if you eat too much protein, some of it will be turned into carbohydrate energy. This was not a problem in 1972, when Atkins first offered his diet to the public. Back then, proteins came with a very different amount of fat, particularly from meat. As our food supply changed, what seemed to be the same plan produced totally different results.

This helps to explain why many people who successfully used those diets years ago have been unsuccessful when they went back and re-tried them now. With the leaner sources of protein available today, those high-protein diets may not produce maximum fat-burning. This hit-or-miss approach keeps your system on the edge between your body's natural fat-burning state and a hunger-inducing sugar-craving state.

- **How does this diet differ from today's popular diets?**

Some diets are aimed at dampening blood-sugar swings, by reducing the worst *glycemic index and glycemic load* carbohydrate offenders. This is helpful for maintaining weight, but at the levels these diets advocate, your brain will continue to crave sugar as an energy source. That makes it difficult to reach a point where you continue to lose weight. This glycemic index is important to understand, but plan to use it once you have reached a goal weight and are keeping your diabetes under dietary control.

- ### What about diets emphasizing dietary fats?

These vary in their emphasis and claims. Diets and other means that greatly reduce dietary fat may actually increase your appetite. This is why research has demonstrated that low-fat dieting is the least effective way to try to lose weight. *There are no magical foods,* or things that will make you lose weight without regard to how much you eat. In this plan, I provide specific recommendations about healthier fats and recommend minimum and maximum amounts.

- ### What about the "epidemic"?

The dual epidemics of type 2 diabetes and obesity are very real and responsible for many health problems around the world. Whether you are reading this because of your own diabetes or because of family members at risk, you will find information regarding food and diet trends that have contributed to this problem. Whether you need to need to follow this plan yourself or not, you will learn which dietary trends you should avoid to protect yourself and those around you.

- ### What background do I have to provide this information?

Following medical school, I focused my career on the prevention of disease. I received a Master of Public Health degree from the Johns Hopkins University while I did my post-graduate medical training, completing the Preventive Medicine residency at the Johns Hopkins University. I then went on to become the Chief Resident of Preventive Medicine at Johns Hopkins, supervising other physicians in the largest nongovernmental preventive medicine program in the nation.

I am Board Certified by the American Board of Preventive Medicine in the specialty of General Preventive Medicine and Public Health, and I am a Fellow of The American College of Preventive Medicine.

I direct weight-loss programs at two clinics in Kansas, one of my own and the other as a volunteer at a charitable Catholic clinic. I recently served as a Fellow and Adjunct Associate Professor in the History of Medicine at the University of Kansas School of Medicine. I have published my method for evaluating the ketogenic nature of food mixtures in the medical literature. I have made presentations concerning obesity and weight-loss at national and international scientific meetings of the following organizations:

- The American College of Preventive Medicine
- The Obesity Society *(formerly North American Association for the Study of Obesity)*
- The American Association for the History of Medicine
- The Indian Health Service of the U.S. Department of the Interior

- **What is preventive medicine?**

Preventive medicine focuses on early interventions and changes to protect your health <u>before</u> serious consequences occur. Unfortunately, the term *"preventive medicine"* is often misused by purveyors of supposedly "magical cures." The true specialty of preventive medicine is one of the recognized branches of medicine in which physicians may train and qualify. Because the current American health care system emphasizes paying practitioners *after* people become ill, there is a serious shortage of doctors willing to undergo the four extra years of training to qualify in this specialty.

- **Is *this* plan to bring your diabetes under control through diet right for you?**

You and your physician are in the best position to answer this. Should you decide it is not right for you, the information in this book should still help you better understand and control your disease.

I have developed a few questions for my patients that may help you decide if this plan is for you.

1. *Are you at least eighteen-years-old?*

This plan was originally developed for adults. Younger people may have special nutritional needs, as well as emotional and family issues requiring additional support. If you intend to use this diet for a younger person, do so with parental support and review that decision with a qualified pediatrician, endocrinologist, or family practitioner before starting.

2. *How much do you need to lose?*

The diet was originally created for people who needed to lose at least twenty pounds. This is not a problem for most type 2 diabetics. However, there are a smaller number of type 2 diabetics who have less of a weight problem than most. Some may not even be overweight by imprecise government body mass index (BMI) standards; yet, they are significantly overweight by evaluating their body fat as a percentage of their total weight. Others may not be overweight at all; yet, their eating habits create the same chaos with their body metabolism.

The good news for type 2 diabetics is that it is not the weight loss alone that brings about change. Most type 2 diabetics experience a dramatic drop in their need for medication and an equally dramatic improvement in control of their diabetes almost as soon as they'd begin to diet, often when they have lost only a few pounds. Therefore, even when weight-loss is not your primary goal, this plan may be useful to you.

3. Are you pregnant or planning to be soon?

Diabetics who become pregnant are a medical challenge. Most will find themselves under the care of an obstetrician who specializes in the endocrinology of pregnancy. If you are pregnant work closely with this specialist. Do not try to lose weight while you are pregnant. Although some animal species carry their young while fasting, people should not. Your developing baby has many nutritional needs and might miss out on some important substances if you diet while pregnant. Often, diabetes becomes more difficult to control during pregnancy. Even women who have not been identified earlier as being diabetic may develop gestational diabetes, a temporary condition that may harm both them and their developing baby and complicate their pregnancy. Those women may be at higher risk for developing type 2 diabetes later in life.

Certainly, if you are pregnant, continue to read the book, but do not start the plan until after you have delivered your baby and are under your physician's monitoring.

If you plan to become pregnant, diet first. Carrying a baby when you have reached a healthy weight and brought your diabetes under better control will be much safer for both you and your child. When on this plan, do not rely on luck for birth control. Diabetes may interfere with the function of your ovaries and your menstrual cycle. Many young women who are overweight and beginning to develop insulin resistance develop polycystic ovary disorder, a condition often characterized by painful and very irregular periods. These women may have difficulty conceiving and family planning may become an afterthought.

Losing weight may improve their condition and, if not careful, they may find themselves pregnant without realizing it. Do not take this risk. The first trimester of pregnancy is extremely important for your developing baby's well-being. Use caution so that you do not become accidentally pregnant while dieting. Once you are at a stable weight and under better control of your diabetes, work with your obstetrician and enjoy a healthier and safer pregnancy for you and your baby.

4. *Are you able to read, write, and understand?*

Since you are reading this book, that answers part of this question, but this plan requires work. I am going to ask you to learn about the foods that you buy and prepare. If you are not sure, you may want to read ahead, *before* you make that commitment.

5. *Do you prepare your own meals?*

This is not a plan for someone who eats out every

meal. If a spouse, companion, or parent prepares your food, be sure that are they willing to assist you in your diabetes control and your weight-loss. If not, are you willing to begin to prepare your own food?

5. Are you medically and psychiatrically stable enough to diet?

Dieting can bring about significant changes, which are usually for the better. However, if you have any condition which requires close monitoring, consider this decision carefully with your personal physician. This is especially true if you take any medication that requires monitoring through blood tests. If you are currently taking any medication to lower your blood sugar, do not try any form of dieting without close monitoring and medication adjustments by your physician. If you have ever been diagnosed with either an eating disorder or bipolar disorder, avoid dieting unless you are working closely with your physician.

If you do not have any problems with any of these issues, you should be able to diet safely, whether with this or any other diet. Of course, there are always exceptions, so check with your physician, if you have questions or doubts about other conditions.

If you passed these "tests," I have a few more questions on the next page. You should try to answer these questions to help you decide if you are motivated enough to begin this plan.

Are You Ready to Begin Controlling Your Health?

1. *Do you have other health problems worsened by your type 2 diabetes and your weight?*
2. *Does your diabetes appear to be worse each year?*
3. *Have you tried the standard diabetic education classes but seem to need more medication with time?*
4. *Has your weight increased as medication has increased?*
5. *Have you ever considered weight-reduction surgery or actually had the surgery but any improvement did not last?*
6. *Are you ready for a change?*

If you answered yes to **any one** of these last six questions, you are definitely ready!

The next chapters will help you understand
why
we are now fighting
epidemics of both overweight and diabetes .

You will learn that you probably did not fail in your previous attempts at controlling your health.
It is likely that your plan failed you.

Chapter 3

Why Prevention?

If you already have diabetes, what good is prevention? "Preventive Medicine" is a broad and well-recognized medical specialty, not the simple catch-phrase that marketers have been using. The understanding that is better to prevent disease, rather than cure it, goes back to ancient times. Efforts at preventing all types of diseases are even older than knowledge of diabetes.

How far back does this knowledge go? Some religious practices mentioned in the Old Testament may lead to better health. The ancient Greeks, generations before Hippocrates, worshipped prevention. The Greeks even had a goddess of prevention and good health, Hygieia.

The ancient Greek physician, Asklepios *(the Romans called him Asclepius)*, was a real physician, but myth turned him into a demi-god, with temples of healing dedicated to him. His daughters represented the two sides of medicine, with three daughters Panakeia, Iaso, and Akeso representing cures and healing, while his daughter Hygieia was the goddess of good health and disease prevention. Our word *hygiene*, describing the science of protecting health, is derived from her name.

Throughout history, teaching how to prevent disease has

been linked to healing. Our common term for healer is "Doctor," which actually describes a learned teacher. For many years, doctors were looked upon as people who could teach others how to remain healthy. Whether what they were actually teaching worked, and whether it was factual, or based on superstition and myth is debatable.

Today, many doctors practice some degree of prevention, but this varies greatly, depending upon their specialty. My specialty, Preventive Medicine and Public Health, is a unique branch of medicine. It has been recognized by the American Medical Association for more than sixty years and requires as many years of post-graduate training as other major medical specialties

Prevention, when it is effective, is more sensible than waiting until a person is ill and then attempting to cure his or her disease. Unfortunately, efforts and money spent on prevention are but a miniscule proportion of the vast amounts spent curing disease. Additionally, many efforts labeled prevention are *not effective* and sometimes turn out to be harmful.

Preventive Medicine is considered to have three components, **primary prevention, secondary prevention,** and **tertiary prevention**. Type 2 diabetes and prevention are linked in each of these three categories.

Primary prevention

Primary prevention can be the most powerful tool we have, but only when it is done effectively. Primary prevention means taking some action so that disease or injury will never occur. Once a preventive measure becomes effective, it is often difficult for people to understand why they are taking that action. A good example is immunization. There is absolutely no question but that immunization is effective in preventing certain disease outbreaks. People who have already suffered through those disease outbreaks understand its value. However, those who never faced the same outbreaks sometimes distrust these efforts. They are fortunate enough to lack first-hand knowledge of what occurred without this important preventive measure.

The weakness with primary prevention is that it may be difficult to understand what works and what does not work. In ancient times, without an understanding of the basis for disease, prevention might have taken the form of superstition. This was innocent enough when it came to wearing amulets to ward off disease, but could do damage when harmful actions were taken to protect the community.

Primary prevention can be subject to the greatest abuse, although superstition in modern times may not involve amulets and spirits. Walk through any large shopping mall and you are likely to see various products and enterprises claiming to improve your health. Theories that have never been shown to prevent disease may be repeated often enough to be believed as if they were fact. Commercial enterprise can capitalize on myths to push products with claims of health benefits, like the legendary "snake-oil" salesman of old.

The reason we have epidemics of obesity and diabetes today can be traced directly to bad decisions by government bodies three decades ago. They took myth and dignified it through regulations and expensive grants. In particular, their ideas about low-fat dieting and the disastrous dietary pyramid were wrong. You may have been following such advice, and seen your diabetes develop or worsen.

Chapter 3   *Why Prevention?*

Additionally, most of the advice offered by the media today is simply wrong. The food industry, which profits from these mistakes, has taken a major role in influencing statements by government agencies which were supposed to be protecting our health. They have even gone as far as infiltrating and influencing professional organizations that make dietary recommendations for the public.

This meddling by those with much to gain commercially has had disastrous results. In fact, many of the claims about healthy foods that people believe today are actually promoting **diabetogenic** foods, foods that are likely to cause diabetes. Companies that produce these foods as well as those who make expensive drugs for diabetes should be delighted.

It is possible to prevent many new cases of diabetes with the proper efforts. To do so, we need to scrap the ineffective recommendations being pushed by people who have built their careers by getting funding for pushing bad advice. Let us go back to what really works. If the government's ideas about prevention were correct, we should have seen improvements since they started pushing bad ideas in the 1970s.

Instead, we have seen the percentage of overweight people quadruple. When this happens, a few years later, expect to see rates for type 2 diabetes follow. So far, diabetes rates have doubled and they are continuing to go higher!

If you or a loved one follow the plan in this book, and you are able to reverse the course of your type 2 diabetes, you will gain an understanding of just how bad the advice you have received in the past may have been. This will provide you a better idea of how to protect yourself and your family.

Secondary prevention

Secondary prevention means controlling the situation before a disease can lead to organ damage and other diseases. In the case of type 2 diabetes, this should mean screening for the early markers for diabetes, to reverse the course of the disease.

This screening can and should be done by your primary care physician, looking for early indications of type 2 diabetes. These indications may include impaired glucose tolerance, often first noticed by patients as midmorning hunger, irritability and a need for snacking. They may include polycystic ovary disorder, often first noticed in young women who have intermittent, painful, or irregular periods. They may include insulin resistance, often detectable by blood tests for circulating natural insulin levels and glycolated hemoglobin (A1c) levels. They may include an expanding waistline, often the first noticeable effect of the metabolic syndrome.

Unfortunately, health insurance companies in the United States, including government Medicare, have made it difficult for doctors to look for these early indications of type 2 diabetes. They discourage laboratory tests that will identify these early stages until someone is clearly diagnosed with a case of diabetes. Due to these restrictions, years go by before someone is diagnosed as diabetic, although they would have benefited from simple dietary changes at an early stage.

Secondary prevention for diabetes should mean detecting and intervening at the earliest possible stage. This is not being done today. Instead, as a nation, we wait until people are at a stage where the prescription of medication can be justified. What do you expect to happen, when the agenda for dietary change is decided by the pill manufacturers and soft-drink companies?

Tertiary prevention

Tertiary prevention can also be good clinical medicine. It involves moderating the course of an established disease to prevent it from causing further harm. In the case of type 2 diabetes, this means preventing complications such as heart attack, stroke, kidney failure, blindness, neuropathy, infections and loss of limbs. These complications are severe end-points for type 2 diabetes, if it is not well-controlled.

Even here, significant improvement is possible for many. Simply giving in and believing that your disease will continue to progress downhill is not an effective solution. Radically changing how your body uses energy may allow natural reversal and healing to take place.

It has been my experience that those I thought would get the least benefit from this plan, those who were already significantly ravaged by disease, sometimes turned out to be those who actually benefited the most. The reason for this paradox seems to be compliance. Many people who diet, whether to lose weight or to control diabetes, often "cheat" occasionally. Unless a person has seen the ravages of diabetes in family or friends, their motivation to take preventive measures often depends on how sick they are already are. Once they see the improvement in their own health, people who had been ill and beaten down by their diabetes, become very, very serious about sticking to this plan 100 percent.

In the past, I have been overweight myself. I have seen the tragedy of diabetes, heart disease, and kidney failure in those close to me. All of these experiences have reinforced my belief that prevention is always better than cure. My life experiences have influenced my choices to pursue disease prevention, whenever possible.

As you read this book, you will have to decide whether this plan is right for you. You and your family will have to decide if you are willing to make significant changes to remain healthy or to regain lost good health. The path is yours to choose.

4

Why are Diabetes and Weight Linked?

The fact that we are now suffering from epidemics of both diabetes and overweight seems absurd. Until recently, the world envied Americans. Statistically, we were taller, thinner, stronger, and had an excellent life expectancy. How did we fall so far, so fast? Why are we turning into a nation of shorter, fatter diabetic people with a decreased lifespan?

Learning the answers to these questions is your key to understanding how choices in your day-to-day activities and food choices have influenced both your weight and your diabetes. You may think that you know many of these answers already, but, if you do, why are you having continuing problems? We will go beyond the shallow and ineffective answers we hear repeatedly in the media.

These problems in America have not occurred because of automobiles, television, or computers. These are usually blamed, and yes, they do contribute to the problem, but the real villain is the manipulation of our food supply on an unprecedented scale. There are several forces behind this. In the 1970s a well meaning but non-medical federal government bureaucracy developed health objectives, which continue to this day. They set important goals encouraging a reduction in dietary fat and an increase in carbohydrates for all Americans. This was the take-off point of the low-fat fad. Government committees responsible for funding the work of university researchers caused scientific dogma to fall into line. Only in the past few years have scientists spoken out strongly, saying these low-fat and high-carbohydrate diets are wrong.

This is a modern version of the fable, *The Emperor's New Clothes.* In that fable, no one wished to be the first to speak out and tell the Emperor that others had made a fool of him. Similarly, scientists who had gone along with our government's edicts about diet were reluctant to point out the problem and appeared to be waiting for someone else to speak out first.

This government-inspired low-fat fad provided a tremendous profit opportunity for the food processing industry. Food processing companies had been creating *faux* or fake foods for years but had to disclose that these foods were imitation. Most consumers looked at these products as second-rate. It costs a lot less to create a fake food than the real product. Now, with the government's blessing, the food industry began to churn out many new versions of these imitation foods coupled with claims that they were healthier! Figure 3-1 on the next page compares what you once got when you asked for cream for your coffee and what the restaurant may give you today. You judge for yourself which product is healthier.

Most Americans today have been so inundated by the combination of advertising claims and well-intentioned advice that they no longer know what to believe. In a society where we are taught to take personal responsibility for our actions, overweight people end up blaming themselves. We find ourselves struggling to lose weight, swimming upstream

---

Figure 3-1

Real Cream   *versus*   **"Creamer"**

Ingredient: Ingredients:

1.   Cream   1.   Water
                        2.   Partially hydrogenated soybean oil
                        3.   Corn syrup solids
                        4.   Sodium caseinate
                        5.   Dipotassium phosphate
                        6.   Sugar
                        7.   Mono and digylcerides
                        8.   Sodium steardyl
                        9.   Lactylate
                        10. Soy lecithin
                        11. Artificial colors
                        12. Artificial flavors

---

against a current of unhealthy food choices.

Ingredients in familiar foods changed. Meals that might not have been fattening before now added on pounds. As people began to get heavier, these same food processors came up with new products to appeal to those who want to slim down. These new, more costly "diet" foods often have just the opposite effect, making you hungrier and causing you to eat more. An intelligent but overweight man sat in my office recently and explained how he had been unable to lose weight. He had tried dieting for years and followed the directions for a particular product. Unfortunately, when he ate this prepared dinner, he was so hungry that he had to have two.

It might be funny, were it not so tragic. Unfortunately, there is nothing funny about the consequences of being overweight. We are not alone in the world. About two-out-of-every three adults in America are now overweight, and the World Health

Organization sees the same problem emerging in the rest of the world. Even in countries traditionally plagued by malnutrition, this modern horror is showing its face. India and China, as they become industrialized, see the same issues. It is ironic that in those places malnutrition and starvation exist side-by-side with obesity.

The reality that being overweight creates many health problems has been recognized since the time of Hippocrates, 2,400 years ago. Today, with a national weight problem greater than any other nation, the United States faces the highest health-care costs in the world. You may not be interested in solving the health problems of our land, but if enough people, just like you, find that they can slim down naturally, it will help. Do it for yourself and you will be setting an example for your family and those around you. Being overweight is not the sole cause of all health problems, but it is a major factor in many, including those listed in Figure 3-2, below.

Figure 3-2

Some Problems Often Worsened or Caused by Overweight

- *Sudden death*
- *Early death*
- *Heart disease*
- *High blood pressure*
- *Stroke*
- *Metabolic syndrome*
- *Diabetes*
- *Kidney disease*
- *Arthritis*

- *Fatigue*
- *Depression*
- *Sexual problems*
- *Skin problems*
- *Snoring*
- *Sleep apnea*
- *Gastro-esophageal reflux*
- *Asthma*
- *and many more*

Diabetes Recovery

This does not answer the question, why are our foods causing us to be fat? The answer is simple. Ask children in the third grade, and they can tell you that if you eat too much, you will get fat. Ask any farmer or rancher how they fatten animals and they will tell you they stuff them with carbohydrates from grain. Japanese Sumo wrestlers were not born fat. Instead, their trainers stuff them with rice carbohydrates to build up fat and *chankonabe* stew for protein to build muscle to move their fatty bulk around. Artificial foods are loaded with both high levels of carbohydrates and appetite-stimulating flavor enhancers to cover the bland tastes of substitute ingredients. Low-fat substitute foods are often very high in sugar.

These changes are well-known to be the best way to *gain* weight, not to lose it. Farmers and ranchers, both ancient and modern, have always known it. Hippocrates taught the ancient world that lesson 2,400 years ago. Yet, the Washington bureaucracy has spent the last three decades pushing these fattening, diabetes-causing diets on the public. All this happened to the delight and profit of both the food processing industry and the pharmaceutical industry. The next chapters will explain how this caused you to add pounds and go on to develop diabetes and how to reverse many of the problems that it has caused for you.

Coincidence?

Do you know do that for much of the past three decades, our food processing companies have been controlled by the tobacco industry. It began as tobacco companies realized fewer people would be smoking cigarettes. The tobacco companies settled on the food industry that would be shielded from change. Trusted and established brands became subsidiaries of big tobacco.

5

How Diabetic Diets Changed

To understand how diabetic diets have changed recently, it is necessary to look back at our understanding of type 2 diabetes over the millennia. Doing this also means understanding some history, not only of medicine, but also of the changing economics of food use.

The diets generally recommended for type 2 diabetics in recent years might have brought horror to the faces of the doctors who did pioneering work in diabetes. Before we had drugs to control diabetes, doctors generally understood that diabetics needed to greatly reduce their intake of sugar and, indeed, of all carbohydrates. How far back this knowledge reaches is shrouded in the distant past of India. Indian medical writings, which appear to be at least 1,200 years old, showed an understanding of the relationship between diet and type 2 diabetes. However, these writings point even further back, to a point where science and legend mingle.

Although other cultures had also recognized diabetes, India is unique. India is considered the birthplace of sugar extraction. Botanists point to the South Seas as the home of the sugarcane plant, which was brought to India 2,700 years ago.

Chapter 5   *How Diabetic Diets Changed*

The process of extracting sugar from the sugarcane plant was developed in India. If you have tried raw sugarcane, you may have had to literally suck the sweetness from this bamboo-like plant.

Extracted sugar was a special treat, reserved for royalty, religious leaders, and the very rich. The process of extracting it was considered a state secret. This enhanced the value of sugar as an expensive spice. Indian physicians quickly noticed that after the introduction of sugar, they had an epidemic of obesity and diabetes among those rich enough to afford this luxury. There is even a legend that Ganeesh, the Hindu god portrayed as half-elephant and half-boy developed "Prameha." Recently, Indian scientists familiar with the ancient literature compared the description of Prameha with a modern definition of type 2 diabetes and found them to be identical.

The legend is that when Ganeesh would travel from village to village, the joyful villagers would always serve him large amounts of rice cakes soaked in sugar syrup, leading to his development of obesity and diabetes. People who have lived in India tell me that this special treat is still consumed during festivals.

Obviously, then, Indian knowledge of type 2 diabetes is ancient. Even the U.S. government commissioned a major study several years ago to identify all the various treatment methods that had been tried for diabetes in ancient India. Knowledge of the relationship between sugar and diabetes traveled slowly, following the path sugar itself traveled.

Because ancient India considered sugar a state secret, knowledge of how to produce it traveled very slowly. When portions of India were conquered by the Persian Empire during an ancient war, the secret of sugar production passed to

Persia. They, too, considered it a valuable commodity and a state secret. Knowledge of sugar production did not spread until 1,200 years ago, when the spread of Islam carried Persian knowledge through much of the Mediterranean. This included the Iberian peninsula, today's Spain and Portugal.

During the sixteenth century, the Portuguese developed mass-scale sugar cultivation and processing. Europeans divided the lands of the new world that they had taken from Native Americans. Portugal recognized that Brazil would be suitable for growing sugarcane on a large scale. To work the land cheaply, they used the trading forts they had already established on the coast of Africa to begin the slave trade and bring enslaved Africans to work the vast plantations.

The other European powers saw the profitability of this venture. They copied the Portuguese and the slave trade grew. Although the cost of transporting sugar was still expensive, the trade of sugar to Europe began to grow. Soon, there were reports from London of sugar-related increases in diabetes.

By the nineteenth century, larger and faster sailing and steam vessels had reduced the cost of transportation and sugar played a larger role in the European diet. When wars and blockades of ports cut off the sugar supply of France, the French government offered a prize for the development of an alternative source of sugar. That led to the cultivation of the sugar beet. Later in the nineteenth century, American companies invented beet harvesting machinery, which brought about further price decreases, and sugar became a common and inexpensive commodity.

Although doctors since ancient times had known about the relationship between diabetes and sugar, it was in the late nineteenth century that much more was understood about the role of dietary carbohydrate and control of diabetes. Dr. Arnaldo Cantani in Italy wrote an important medical book about balancing food intake to control obesity and diabetes during the 1870s. Dr. Wilhelm Ebstein carried this work farther in Germany in the 1880s. These diets emphasized significant avoidance of carbohydrates, with a corresponding increase in the amount of dietary energy obtained from fat. Similar dietary therapy remained the mainstay for type 2 diabetes for decades.

In 1922, Doctors Frederick Banting and Charles Best of Toronto were responsible for the discovery of insulin. This was an important step forward and insulin therapy was quickly embraced. It was, and still is, the basic therapy for type 1 diabetes. However, type 2 diabetics would continue to attempt to be controlled through dietary therapy and turn to insulin use only if they were unable to control their condition by diet alone. Over the years, many variations of insulin therapy were developed. Newer insulins, with different patterns of timing, helped diabetics bring better control over their sugar levels while attempting to avoid dangerous hypoglycemic or low-sugar episodes. Type 2 diabetics under poor control were often reluctant to begin the needle use, which insulin therapy required.

The recognition that certain types of drugs changed the body's response to sugar metabolism led to the development of oral therapy, pills for diabetes, by the 1970's. These were considered a breakthrough, giving type 2 diabetics an alternative to insulin when diet alone failed them. Unfortunately, that was when dietary therapy started to go wrong. Prior to that, diabetic diets were extremely low in carbohydrates of all forms and instead, used increased amounts of fat for an energy source. Suddenly, dietary recommendations for diabetics changed.

The reasons for the shift away from fat-balanced diets as a primary energy source were twofold. First, there was the fear of fat. Some of this fear was perfectly rational while some of it was highly irrational. Tthere was an erroneous belief by some scientists was that dietary fat was the primary cause of cholesterol imbalance, obesity and heart disease in everyone. This was only partially true, because they used data to "prove" this idea solely from societies with high sugar consumption. As an example, In the United States today, we consume well over 100 pounds of sugar a year per person. This is about <u>thirty times</u> the amount per person that Americans used when our nation was founded.

What was ignored was the data for societies where large amounts of sugar and other carbohydrates were not consumed. In those situations, the increased use of fat did not lead to disease. By concentrating only on sugar metabolism and ignoring the natural mechanism for fat metabolism, the drew erroneous conclusions. This led to the anti-fat hysteria and the false belief that that all fats were bad.

It is this high sugar consumption that leads to increased insulin output, which both signals the body to store fat, even creating new fat when a low-fat diet is followed. This leads to the insulin resistance, which worsens the cycle of type 2 diabetes. As cells become more and more resistant to insulin, the pancreas is stressed to produce even more insulin. Eventually, this stress wears the pancreas out, resulting in less insulin production and worsening the need for diabetic medication.

The other reason for the shift away from fat-centered diets to carbohydrate-centered diets has to do with the introduction of oral anti-diabetic medication itself. Using pills, it is far more difficult to target an exact amount of medicine needed to control blood sugar. Since the use of insulin began, doctors have attempted to determine a precise amount needed for a particular patient. While this insulin strategy is not always perfect, it is impossible when using pills. Insulin doses can easily be varied by minute amounts, but pills cannot.

Both insulin and most oral diabetic medication can cause dangerous hypoglycemic episodes, where the medication causes blood sugar to go too low. This dangerous condition can cause strokes and heart attacks by depriving body tissue of any nutrition. Although long-recognized with diabetics using insulin, it is a far greater danger when using pills.

This problem with hypoglycemia was quickly recognized as a danger when pills were introduced. As an "answer" to prevent this dangerous condition, dietitians were taught to instruct diabetic patients to eat more carbohydrates. This is taught as if it were a good thing. In fact, it is a safety measure, to protect these individuals from these hypoglycemic episodes <u>caused by</u> their medication. This puts you, the diabetic, in a double-bind. Too little carbohydrate can result in dangerous hypoglycemia. Too much carbohydrate means higher sugar levels, prompting your doctor to increase medication levels. The results can be a vicious cycle, chasing ever-elusive control of diabetes, while moving to more expensive and more powerful medication.

A number of years ago, health authorities in the United States and Europe reasoned that bringing sugar levels down to normal in diabetics would decrease the damage that causes stroke, heart attack, blindness, kidney failure, neuropathy and other illnesses. They were totally correct in what they tried to do, but were mistaken in how they tried to do it. Major research trials attempted to achieve "perfect" control of blood sugar with ever-increasing doses of diabetic medication.

The results of their research were alarming. Because they were using medication rather than strictly dietary methods, more people had strokes or died as a result of this "therapy."

Finally, they stopped their research. In retrospect, they realized that attempting to bring diabetics into a normal sugar range when using pills put more people at risk for hypoglycemia and led to increased deaths from strokes. On the other hand, the people they did not kill with this strategy seemed to do better overall. The underlying idea of bringing sugar under better control was correct, but was the strategy of doing that with ever-increasing doses of pills was the wrong method!

Recognizing their mistake, rather than reducing the ever-increasing dependence on pills to control diabetes, they changed their goals. Instead of attempting to bring people to normal levels of blood sugar, they first created a dual standard and more recently have weakened their standard. What that means is that they now never attempt to get diabetics to return to normal. Instead, they have deliberately set the desired goals for diabetics more loosely. What has this accomplished? At best, therapy which does not truly bring sugar levels to a normal state may slow the progress of other medical conditions due to diabetes, but will not prevent all the damage.

On the other hand, people successfully using diet alone have been shown to completely come off diabetic medication with good control of blood sugar levels. This eliminates the danger reducing sugar so that further damage to other organs of the body can be stopped.

Will a strictly dietary approach work for everyone? No, but it may benefit the majority of type 2 diabetics. After many years of high sugar levels and insulin resistance, some diabetics will go on to develop severe insulin insufficiency. That is, their pancreas becomes worn out from overuse. In the earlier stages of diabetes, reversibility is easier. Nevertheless, I have seen diabetics who were on a combination of insulin and pills for over a decade learn how to bring their sugar under excellent control strictly by diet.

Why haven't you been told this before? The reasons are economic, not medical. Diabetes today is a multi-billion dollar business. Many experts on diabetes receive money from drug companies. Researchers receive grant money to continue their work when they are developing drugs with billion dollar potential. Publications and media receive hundreds of millions in advertising revenue from the makers and suppliers of diabetes drugs and equipment. If you watched television today, how many commercials did you see for diabetes drugs or supplies? Scientific publications try to have authors disclose conflicts of interest, but things slip through.

In recent years, there has been an even worse trend in misinforming both the public and health professionals. Recently, I read a "puff piece" in my local newspaper. It was one of those so-called news items that actually came from a press release from a publicity agent. It quoted a supposed authority, reassuring the public that there was *"no relationship between the consumption of sugar and the development of diabetes."* When I checked, I discovered that the expert quoted was a spokesperson for a professional organization, which sets standards used by dietitians. I was baffled by this strange position until I noticed the fine print on the organization's website. It stated that their officially sanctioned statements were "*developed jointly with industry.*" Later, a leading medical journal article showed that this organization actually received hundreds of thousands of dollars each year from a soft-drink manufacturer!

Recently, an important organization representing family physicians agreed to take soft-drink money. Some physicians quit this organization in protest, but there are many other organizations not wanting to raise their dues during hard economic times. The temptation to accept these "gifts" is an easy way for publicists to influence both public and professional thinking in dangerous ways.

You may ask an apparent question. *If old-fashioned dietary control is possible, why didn't more people stick to the old method?* The answer is that they did not have all the tools we have today, which make success far more likely. Dietary control of diabetes today can be far more accurate, thanks to two developments that most diabetics are already familiar with and should be using regularly.

One is the glycoscylated or glycated hemoglobin test, more commonly known as the hemoglobin A1c test. This test shows what your average blood sugar was in the two-to-three months preceding the test. This is extremely meaningful. Before the development of this test, doctors had to rely upon the occasional fasting blood sugar levels, taken early in the morning. Unfortunately, particularly in the earlier stages of diabetes, these may appear normal for years while your blood sugar is actually taking wild high and low swings and damaging your heart and kidneys. Perhaps you know someone whose diabetes was not diagnosed until after they had a heart attack or kidney failure. A1c is a highly reliable way to determine your average reading. It registers the percentage of red blood cells that have been changed by blood sugar. The only time it is not considered accurate is when a person also has another problem with their blood. Fasting blood sugar only shows the level of your blood sugar at one particular instant, although there is a variation throughout the day. The variation of blood sugar during the day reflects your dietary habits, your body's insulin resistance, and your ability to produce insulin. By giving you an average reading, A1c provides a glimpse of the overall picture.

The second development has been the invention and widespread use of home-glucose-monitoring equipment. Every diabetic should have this. Some doctors and insurance companies would rather limit these to the most severe cases, but they allow earlier control of diabetes, so that they do not progress to severe cases. When using dietary control, these meters serve as a feedback mechanism to the diabetic. You can easily see the effect of particular food on your control. Newer, more accurate meters have become available. Most of these newer models require only a fraction of the blood sample that the earlier meters required. This allows the diabetic to take a sample from a reasonably non-painful spot rather than a fingertip.

Another useful tool is the algorithm, which I developed to estimate the mixture of food required to put you in a fat-burning state. Combined together with the suggestions in this book, you and your doctor can see the impact of dietary control on improving the status of your diabetes and reducing or eliminating your diabetic medication.

Will you succeed? I believe so. If you are looking for an answer by reading this book, you may have the determination to take the steps needed to reverse your disease. The majority of diabetics I have seen using this plan have done just that.

There are exceptions. This diet will greatly reduce the sugar-caused craving to eat more than you need. That craving is actually a useful bodily mechanism to make you put on fat when the food supply is abundant, so that you can survive by burning off that fat during lean times. Since we do not live in that type of agricultural world anymore, having that reading constantly turned on creates a biologic mechanism that was overemphasizing your hunger in the past. This led to overeating, being overweight and developing type 2 diabetes.

Many people also overeat for emotional reasons. Interestingly, when your body is sugar-craving, anxiety triggers are turned on and when you satisfy those triggers by eating, you temporarily feel calm. This leads to a learned response, where you often may eat whenever you are upset. Although this is not actual hunger, it stimulates you the same way. For this reason, support and learning new responses are helpful for many people losing weight. At the extreme level, people who succumb to this are sometimes diagnosed with a binge eating disorder. Although this pattern may be well established, they too can be helped by a diet that takes away the underlying physiologic drive to overeat.

People that try to "mix and match" therapies will not respond well to dietary therapy. The plan in this book needs to be followed carefully, with your doctor's approval and supervision. Some people get advice from many, including professionals, acquaintances and self-styled Internet gurus. In an effort to please everyone, they may try a little bit of this and a little bit of that. That is not going to work.

Finally, there are a smaller percentage of poorly controlled type 2 diabetics who have gone from the classic insulin resistance to severe insulin insufficiency. Biologically, at that point, they resemble type 1 diabetics, in that their pancreas can no longer do its job. Diet alone may not be enough in this case. However, as I explained earlier, I have seen people who were very far along in their disease show remarkable improvement. Perhaps it is the impact of removing the constant battering that their metabolic control mechanisms had suffered, which allowed healing to take place.

6

How Food Changes You

Why do faux foods make you gain weight and develop type 2 diabetes? Three important factors have come together. These are the following:

1. Actual Food Content
2. Appetite stimulants
3. Portion size

The switch from naturally balanced food products to low-fat carbohydrate-rich foods is the number one villain in this story. Diabetics know that *insulin* has a role in controlling their blood

Figure 6.1	
Insulin	***Glucagon***

- *Increases when sugar in blood is high*
- *Signals body to use sugar*
- *Signals body to store energy*
- *Signals body that excess sugar is to be stored as fat*

- *Increases when sugar in blood is low*
- *Signals body that energy is needed*
- *Signals body to release stored energy*
- *Signals body to convert fat to ketones*

sugar, but not everyone understands that **glucagon**, insulin's balancing companion, is designed to work together with insulin, controlling your energy balance.

Both insulin and glucagon are produced in adjacent cells of your pancreas and have opposite effects. Working as a team, they control the ebb and flow of energy in your body, allowing all of your cells to get the energy they need, whether that energy comes from the food you recently ate or from stored energy, coming from food you ate at an earlier time.

Your body stores its energy in two ways. One way is to create a starch called *glycogen* for short-term energy. Consider it your "between meals" energy source. Another way is to create fat for long-term energy. Consider fat your "off season" energy source. It works fine in nature. Bears eat ravenously during the summer and fall, loading up on carbohydrates, which get turned into fat. They rely on the insulin they produce to turn this excess energy into stored energy. During their off season, they hibernate and their body switches over to burning their stored fat.

People, on the other hand, have gotten very good at storing food supplies for their off season. Today, with most of us shopping at supermarkets, we forget what a short harvest season our ancestors had.

If we eat like bears preparing for winter but never hibernate, we will grow fat. It goes back to that third-grade knowledge. If we eat more than we need, we will get fat. If we want to lose weight, like the bear, we must eat less than we need so our bodies burn up our stored energy.

We wish it were that simple. All we would have to do would be to eat less. That is what people keep telling us, then condemn us as morally weak when we cannot lose. Research scientists can easily demonstrate how almost any diet works, if people behaved like test mice in cages. Unfortunately, that is the extent of the supposed successful testing of many diets.

Pay a group of college women to try out a diet in a locked dormitory during a school break and they will lose weight. The true test of a diet should be whether the weight loss holds true once

Figure 6-2

you remove the bars from the cage or the lock from the kitchen.

If a diet leaves you constantly hungry, remove the restraints and, like our little mouse, you will want to eat more. If you are very determined, you may lose weight but will probably hate every moment of that diet. An effective diet must do more. A diet that works must get your body to burn fat yet make you feel that you have had enough. Hippocrates described the first such diet and others through the ages have re-discovered the secret. The secret, it turns out, is not a secret at all.

Since your body can only burn two types of energy, everything that you eat gets turned into

Figure 6-3

one of these two fuels. They are either sugar, in the form of *glucose*, or fat, turned into a form called *ketones*. Almost every cell in your body can use either one, but like a dual-fueled vehicle or building, adjustments must be made. Cars equipped to run on either gasoline or *E85* ethanol have sensors and computer programs to decide how to adjust the engine based on what fuel mix is running. You, too, have a complex system, with many signal pathways and transmitters, but at the heart of it all is that insulin-glucagon balance.

Initially, when we are eating large amounts of carbohydrate, our brains always cry out for sugar. When we starve or fast, our muscles switch to burning fat and our body keeps our brain pumped up on sugar. We feel hungry and irritable because we know we are low on energy. That can only last a day or two, because that sugar is coming from our stored up glycogen, our between meals energy supply. After a day or two, as we run very low on sugar, our brains give in and switch to burning fat. Now, we have an ample supply of energy. Although we will be missing other nutrients, we have enough energy for several months. Our hunger is reduced.

This is a tricky time for diabetics who are on medication. Most diabetics have already received proper instruction about the need to reduce or totally stop diabetic medication at times they reduce their food intake or increase their energy use through exercise. At least, they should have received that instruction. I have met a number of diabetics who say they were never instructed in this important area. Perhaps they forgot it, or perhaps everyone in the system thought someone else had told them.

If you were never instructed about when to hold medication, or do not remember it, go get that instruction now. Whether you decide to follow this plan or not, knowing when to hold off on taking medication is vital and may save you from serious harm. If you fast or reduce your energy intake, continuing most diabetic medication without change will cause your blood sugar to go too low. The resulting hypoglycemic episode will be frightening and may lead to devastating consequences, such as a stroke.

In fact, burning fat has other effects. Once we get over the initial discomfort of making the change, we may actually feel better and be able to think more clearly. For some people suffering from a seizure disorder, their brains quiet down and seizures decrease or disappear. A pure fast brings about profound changes in brain chemistry. These bring about changes that have been understood in differing cultures and civilizations, for millennia. You do not need to understand biochemistry to understand the inner peace and mental tranquility that many have reported. Here are some examples:

Recall that:

- *Jesus went to the desert and fasted (for forty days)*
- *Old Testament prophets fasted*
- *Native Americans fasted*
- *Mystics in India fasted*

All experienced a clarity of thought and peace during this religious or mystic experience. Fasting, in many cultures, seems to be a path to inner peace and enlightenment.

Almost a century ago, physicians researched this phenomena and discovered that it was the condition of *ketosis,* the fat-burning state associated with finding ketones in the bloodstream, that caused the powerful brain changes that suppressed seizures. With that knowledge, they were able to duplicate the seizure suppression of fasting while allowing patients to still eat. Today, there are many powerful medications that can be used to treat those seizure disorders. However, dietary treatment is still used occasionally today, especially in children who have not been helped by medicines or surgery. It is used infrequently, because it is difficult to follow, requiring a diet of little except fat or oil. However, because it is so effective, researchers conducted a large clinical trial in 2008, once again proving the validity of that older discovery from the 1920s.

It was this knowledge that allowed me to go one step further, in creating a diet for weight-loss. I found that the mathematical formula developed years ago through research on the therapeutic "ketogenic diet" could be adapted to weight-loss dieting. Ketosis signals fat burning and suppresses hunger, but modern weight-loss diets that stressed ketosis were hit or miss. Most stressed carbohydrate reduction or substituted proteins for carbohydrates, and they worked for some but not for others. I know that all too well, because I gained more than fifty unwanted pounds following all the supposed healthy eating recommendations. Those "recommended" diets did nothing for me, which is why I searched for and developed a better way.

On the one hand, eating a diet of almost pure fat would definitely produce ketosis. On the other hand, eating nothing at all would also definitely produce ketosis. I found that the formula developed long ago could be mathematically modified to predict the points in between. The computer model that resulted showed when weight-reduction diets were likely to produce ketosis and when they were not. Diets that are low in calories but just on the edge of ketosis, keep you in constant turmoil. A diet that fails to keep you in fat burning leaves your brain crying out for sugar and you constantly may feel hungry. The computer model demonstrated how all diets could be ketogenic if their total calories were but a tiny fraction of your daily needs.

Diets that were low in their amount of fat but high in carbohydrate quickly stopped being ketogenic as soon as calories increased slightly. Diets that were low in carbohydrate and high in protein could increase calories a little, but they too stopped producing ketosis at some point. This made sense, since the protein you eat gets broken down into amino acids.

Some amino acids get used as replacement building blocks in your tissues, while the remainder get used as energy. Since energy comes from either sugar or fat, amino acids break down to one or the other. That means that too much protein may produce enough sugar to stop ketosis.

A diet low in carbohydrate, moderate in protein and the balance of its energy coming from fat can stay ketogenic from starvation levels all the way up to fully meeting your daily energy requirements. At the higher energy levels, such a diet would be very high in fat, just like the diet still prescribed for those children having seizures, a regimen that is difficult to follow.

Physicians try to follow the rule *"Primum non nocere,"* meaning *"First, do no harm."* For that reason, I took a conservative approach and have set some additional limits. I set an upper limit for fat at less than 70 grams per day, which is about the amount of fat someone who was not losing weight would get from a low-fat diet recommended by heart disease advocates. I set a lower limit for protein of about 40 grams of per day for most people, an adequate amount for healthy adults. The resultant graph is shown in Figure 6.4.

The fat-centered diet line remains high and stays above the dotted line while the other two fall rapidly and lose their fat-burning potential. The filled in area represents what I consider the optimum starting point for most dieters. Although this is what I recommend, I have had people try for less. Once they sense what works for them, people do experiment. My recommendation is conservative and can produce a steady

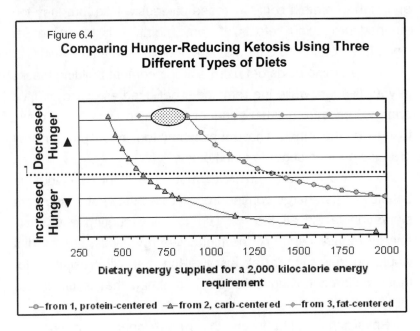

Figure 6.4
Comparing Hunger-Reducing Ketosis Using Three Different Types of Diets

average weight loss of about two pounds (or about one kilo) a week over the long term.

Once you are in a fat-burning mode, everything changes. Since your sugar level is no longer elevated, the beta-cells of your pancreas can rest. The insulin receptors throughout your body are no longer being pushed by constant excess insulin levels, and they, too, begin to rest. How much healing can take place depends on how far you have gone, and how much damage has been created. If you can keep that sugar level in control, you will find remarkable changes. This, of course, requires you to watch your blood glucose through your home-monitoring device. This rest period is quickly evident. The biological markers for inflammation of your blood vessels begin to return to normal. Your liver, instead of creating fat from carbohydrate and sending it to storage, now is using that stored fat to turn into energy. You have reversed the energy flow that was leading to a high risk for heart attack and stroke.

In the past, diabetics were often taught to fear the fat-burning state of ketosis. Before there were devices to monitor your glucose at home, insulin-dependent diabetics had to rely upon urine testing to determine whether their insulin was keeping them in good control. Unlike the meters of today, which are highly accurate, urine tests for sugar are often very inaccurate. Yet, they were the best technology available for home-monitoring. Urine testing for sugar does not detect anything until blood sugar is highly out of control. Under extreme conditions, such a diabetic might have had the combination of a high blood sugar but no energy reaching their cells. In such a case, their body would sense starvation and switched to burning ketones. This was often termed "Starving in the midst of plenty." This combination would signify that a diabetic's disease was so out of control that they needed to be hospitalized as a medical emergency. The urine testing strip for sugar also contained a second testing strip for ketosis. The combination of extremely high blood sugar, ketosis, strong metabolic acidosis and a *hyper-osmolar state*, meaning that their blood was thick with sugar, was extremely dangerous. Therefore lacking other information, even a hint of ketosis was treated as a "panic value," where the laboratory would make an emergency call to a doctor.

This is not the case with someone who is deliberately dieting. In this situation, ketosis is the normal physiologic condition. If blood sugar remains in the normal range, ketosis while dieting should not be feared by a type 2 diabetic. Without the high sugar level, there will not be the dangerous hyper-osmolar state, with the blood becoming heavy from its high sugar content. Ketones represent fat, which is acidic. Therefore, with most energy coming from fat, the body will have to adjust to this extra acid. This will temporarily create a mild acidic condition in the blood, called *metabolic acidosis*, but should be within the range that the body can adjust for. As long as you remain in the state, your body will have a chance to create its own bicarbonate buffers and return the pH level of the blood to a comfortable state This should not be a problem and the process can easily be speeded up by the addition of some mild bicarbonate to the diet. The key difference here, is that a modern diabetic is doing close home-monitoring. Therefore, he or she knows that blood sugar is in a normal or near-normal range.

Those who follow this diet successfully take a few weeks to get the hang of it and understand how their body reacts. Some people will reduce their diet even more, realizing that they can quicken their weight loss. Most patients add exercise, which I heartily recommend. Hippocrates, too, recommended increased exercise, in his *Method of Losing or Gaining Weight.* Exercise helps everyone and you should exercise, <u>to the extent that you are able</u>.

Unfortunately, some diets use the excuse that their diet <u>only</u> works if you exercise. That is a case of shifting blame to the victim. Let's face it, telling a middle-aged office worker carrying sixty or seventy extra pounds to get into sweats and follow the twenty-something exercise leader at a health club may be futile. Some people will not even go to the gym because they suffer from self-loathing as a result of being overweight and dread being seen in gym clothing. Some brave souls try to keep up, overdoing it and harming themselves.

Try to visualize that spandex-clad instructor carrying the equivalent of your extra weight in a backpack. That is the exercise you are already doing simply going through your daily activities. Do not be shamed into believing you must exercise beyond your means. Instead, start out gradually. For my heaviest dieters, this can mean just walking a little farther each day or going to a "Y" with a pool and joining a water-exercise group. Play a little more with your children, nieces and nephews or grandkids. Be reasonable and work up to the tougher stuff as you lose weight. Let your own body be your guide.

Increasing your activity level through a regular exercise regimen might mean that your loss will be greater than two pounds a week. Either way, be patient. Remember, a loss of two pounds a week, means you can lose a hundred pounds in less than a year.

Have you had enough of charts and graphs? You may be

turning pages and asking what the "magic formula" is. Everyone's needs differ, but a good starting point is based on considering a person who needs 2,000 kilocalories of energy each day. This should work well to start for most people but individual adjustment may be needed for some.

Think of this **60-40-10** mix as a starting point. If you burn about 2,000 calories each day, this mixture should provide about 37 percent of your energy needs, maintain a moderate-to-strong state of fat-burning and result in about a two pound weight loss each week. Try to keep your fat consumption up, eating at least 60 grams each day, but try to not go over 70 grams. Special instructions will be given later for those who must restrict their fat intake. Protein should be kept to around 40 grams each day, but may be increased slightly if you decrease your carbohydrate below the 10 grams allowed each day. If you do this, you may substitute 2½ grams of protein for each gram of carbohydrate less than the 10 grams allowed. Although there are minimum "essential" fats and protein needs in anyone's diet, there is no such thing as an essential need for carbohydrates. The carbohydrate allowance can go lower, but you want to include some green leafy vegetables and other foods containing small amounts of carbohydrate each day .

Since these amounts are listed in grams, how do you know what food actually contains? There are several ways to get this information as you select foods. First, using the recipes in this book, you will find estimated counts with each recipe. If you are obtaining recipes from cookbooks or the Internet, look for recipes that include such information. Packaged foods include this information as part of their food labeling. Fresh meat, poultry, seafood, and vegetables do not come with product labels, although some markets do provide information sheets.

For the rest, use either any standard guidebook that you want to purchase or check the Internet. How to use a nutritional label is explained later in the chapter on shopping. The next chapter suggests how to prepare before starting your diet.

Figure 5-5	**The 60-40-10 Daily Plan**
Fat	**60 grams** *(but not more than 70)*
Protein	**40 grams** *(up to 65 if carbohydrates are cut)*
Carbohydrate	**10 grams** *(or less if you want more protein)*

7

Getting Ready

Congratulations! Since you have gotten this far, you are preparing to start this plan. Take the time to get ready before starting. Meet with the provider who monitors your diabetes to agree on a plan. You must do three things, now. First, set a weight-loss goal. Next, you and your doctor must plan how you will monitor your glucose and reduce your medication before starting. Finally, go shopping for the food and supplies you will need to begin the plan.

It is likely that you will see your recovery from diabetes begin almost as soon as you start this plan. Setting your weight-loss goal first helps you have dual goals, which can improve your direction and purpose. Do not be afraid of doing this, because this diet can really work if you apply it!

Setting your weight-goal realistically is important. If you are reluctant to set a goal because of previous failures, remember that you did not fail before, your diet failed you! The next page provides a body-mass-index (BMI) chart. BMI is important for researchers and statisticians but is not the best way for you to set your personalized goal. The boxes on the next few pages will help explain why BMI is imperfect and explain other ways to set a goal.

Continued on page 68

Finding your BMI Category

Note: BMI treats men and women equally.

Height	Under-weight	Normal		Overweight		Obese		Extremely Obese
	Less than	From	To	From	To	From	To	More than
BMI	**18.5**	**18.5**	**24.9**	**25**	**29.9**	**30**	**39.9**	**39.9**
			Body Weight in pounds					
4' 11"	92	92	123	124	147	148	197	197
5'	95	95	127	128	152	153	203	203
5' 1"	98	98	131	132	157	158	210	210
5' 2"	101	101	135	136	163	164	217	217
5' 3"	105	105	140	141	168	169	224	224
5' 4"	108	108	144	145	173	174	231	231
5' 5"	111	111	149	150	179	180	239	239
5' 6"	115	115	154	155	185	186	246	246
5' 7"	118	118	158	159	190	191	254	254
5' 8"	122	122	163	164	196	197	261	261
5' 9"	125	125	168	169	202	203	269	269
5' 10"	129	129	173	174	208	209	277	277
5' 11"	133	133	178	179	214	215	285	285
6'	137	137	183	184	220	221	293	293
6' 1"	140	140	188	189	226	227	301	301
6' 2"	144	144	193	194	232	233	310	310
6' 3"	148	148	199	200	239	240	318	318
6' 4"	152	152	204	205	245	246	327	327

If you want to know your exact BMI, you can use an Internet calculator provided by The National Institute of Health at http://www.nhlbisupport.com/bmi/bmicalc.htm

Pitfalls using BMI

BMI is a statistical starting point, not an individual evaluation. It is totally inadequate for many.

Consider a woman who is 5 feet 3 inches tall. Her "healthy" BMI would place her weight between 105 and 140 pounds, what she weighed in high school. However, her bones and muscles have remodeled to carry her extra weight. At 280 pounds, she now has 140 pounds of fat, exactly half of her weight. The remaining 140 pounds represents her "lean body mass" and is composed of everything that is not fat.

BMI has created an impossible goal for her, recommending she lose at least 140 pounds to be "healthy." Nobody can live without some body fat. Young women are healthy when they have about 19 to 22 percent of their body weight in fat, but this percentage increases with age. Only an extremely fit athlete, might go a few points lower.

Using a measured body fat percentage, a realistic goal for this woman would be between 173 and 179 pounds. Later, as her body has remodeled at a lower weight, she can be rechecked and a lower goal might then be possible.

You probably have been told what your *"ideal weight"* should be based on BMI, but that is just a statistical guess based solely on your height. It is likely that your physician recommended a "healthy weight" for you based on the BMI, but this can lead to serious problems. If you have been seriously overweight for many years, your bone and muscle mass has grown to carry that weight. Attempting to reach an "ideal weight" based solely on BMI could result in a goal that is dangerously underweight.

Rather than BMI alone, use either one of these two factors in deciding what your goal should be. Even better, use them together. First, consider your weight history, by asking yourself what you weighed at various points in your life and what you would like to get back to. Next, measure your percentage of body fat to find your healthiest weight. There are many ways to determine that percentage, even if you are doing this by yourself at home.

Once you estimate how much fat is on your body now, you can determine what your weight should be with a healthy amount of body fat. After determining your body fat, you can calculate *"lean body mass"*, which means how much your body would weigh with no fat. Next, using a percentage of body fat appropriate for your age and sex, a reasonable weight goal can be estimated. More information on how to do this is available on-line at *www.HippocraticDiet.com*. A physician, nurse or a well-trained instructor at a local gym may be able to assist you in this. In addition to weight, set other personal goals that you would like to reach. This could be a clothing size, waist measurement, or something personally meaningful.

Next, develop a medication and monitoring plan with your physician. **This is a critical step for all diabetics.** If you have

Continued on page 70

Measuring your Body Fat

There are several easy ways to measure your body fat. Two of these can be done in the privacy of your own home.

Inexpensive bathroom scales that use electrical impedance to calculate body fat actually work. They are usually accurate to within a few percentage points, although the numbers they produce will vary somewhat during the day.

Skin calipers can be purchased for a few dollars at both sporting and medical supply stores. Skin calipers are used to measure the thickness of a pinch of your skin. Professionals measure at seven spots and use a computer to perform complex calculations. Home calipers use a single measure to do the same thing. That is often close enough for you, but be sure that your caliper comes with instructions for home use.

One weakness of the caliper method is that it will underestimate your body fat when you have a large waistline. The caliper is measuring the thickness of the fat layer immediately under your skin. The most dangerous form of fat, which is common in diabetics, is omental fat or internal belly fat, which is actually deposited inside your abdominal cavity. That is why using a waistline measurement as a goal is another important tool.

DEXA is a tool available in the X-ray department of some medical centers that gives an accurate assessment. Unfortunately, medical insurance will usually not pay for its use.

not yet been started on medication, you are at an advantage. Your plan should consist of having your physician measure your hemoglobin A1c shortly before beginning this program and monitoring your glucose levels at home. However, if you are on medication, you must be in synchronization with your physician. Ideally, your physician or other practitioner has clearly spelled out to you those times when you must hold medication. As an example, if you are fasting for a medical test or if you change your exercise pattern, you should have been taught enough to know about checking your sugar level and withholding medication when necessary. Although that is ideal, I have found that many patients have never received this type of counseling.

If you have not been instructed about when to hold medication, stop right here. Do not begin this plan without further discussion with your medical provider, the one who is prescribing the medication for your diabetes. When you initiate your diet, you will do little to raise your blood sugar at all. Because of this, your usual dose of diabetic medication may cause dangerous hypoglycemic episodes. This should not be a time for either compromise or do-it-yourself solutions.

You will need to monitor your blood sugar reliably. Four times a day is preferred and be sure you write it down. Later in this book, we will show you a convenient way to monitor all of your activity. This will help you in controlling your sugar while you lose weight.

How much should you cut back or eliminate your medication? This <u>must be determined by your medical provider</u>. I usually have patients who are on one or two diabetic medications temporarily hold them completely. Once they initiate their diet with a partial fast, they may see slightly elevated blood sugars, which tend to revert to a normal range as their bodies burn up their stored sugar reserves. If they have been on a large doses of more medication, I will prescribe or have them continue a small to moderate dose of Metformin. This will allow the insulin that they normally produce to be more effective in overcoming insulin resistance without a high danger of hypoglycemic reaction.

This discussion is a generalization, and needs to be modified to meet your individual needs by your physician or provider, who hopefully understands the physiology of fasting and dieting. Whatever you do, if you cannot control your diabetes without continued high doses of medication, this diet is not going to be appropriate for you. You should continue to read this book, as you may learn things which will still be helpful and useful to you, but you might find your diabetes too advanced to completely control with this plan.

The good news is that most type 2 diabetics are able to regain control of their blood sugar just on this diet. I have seen a few people fail. The ones that fail were typically on four or five medications and had fasting blood sugar of 300 to 400 despite all medications prescribed by their endocrinologist.

I have also cautioned people not to use this diet if they were episodic binge eaters or did not take responsibility for remaining on a diet. There are people who have emotional issues that prevent them from committing to a course of action. The person who tries to please everyone may fail. Since this plan differs from others, some people will get conflicting advice from both professionals and non-professionals. In an attempt to compromise and please everyone, they generally will please no one and may harm themselves. One dangerous example is the person who does not wish to displease his or her physician by stopping a medication but wants to follow this plan. That person may do himself or herself great harm.

If those examples do not describe you, you will probably do well. Be sure that your physician is willing to take your phone calls or have his or her nurse follow you. I generally will see my patients every few days when they begin this plan. I tell diabetics not to be concerned if they see a glucose level of 150 or 160 for a few days. For most of them, this will revert to normal values rapidly. Higher levels might require adding or increasing Metformin. Still higher levels may indicate someone who would have further difficulty and is not appropriate for strict dietary control without additional medication.

The important issue is maintaining communication with your physician, particularly in the first few weeks. After three months on this plan, be sure to have your A1c repeated. I have seen many people who had an A1c between 7.0 and 10.0 on medication drop to an A1c level between 5.5 and 6.2 off medication. That change is important, because it shows a tremendous improvement in average blood sugar, which in turn can lead to improvements in all of the medical conditions caused by type 2 diabetes.

Next, before beginning, clean your cupboard and go shopping. If you live alone, get rid of all the foods that either made you fat or diabetic. If you live with others, think about separating some of your food items. Later, your family or companions may want some of the foods you will be preparing, but for now, do not let their preferences influence what you put into your body.

The next pages have two lists of foods, some to clean out and others to stock. Get these basic items to stock for your cupboard, since they are foods that you will use in your diet

Continued on page 75

Foods to Clear Out

- *Sugar, honey, corn syrup, maple syrup, and other sugary syrups*
- *Flour, corn meal, oatmeal, breakfast cereals and other grain products*
- *Potatoes, rice, peas, beans, spaghetti, noodles, pasta, and other starchy foods*
- *Bread, croutons, crackers, cookies, cakes, muffins, donuts, and other baked goods*
- *Soft drinks, except calorie-free products*
- *Alcoholic beverages*
- *Salad dressing containing carbohydrate or MSG (as most do)*
- *All fruit drinks and sugary fruits*
- *All soups, unless MSG-free (not "No added MSG)*
- *Dessert mixes, unless sugar-free*
- *Processed meats unless MSG-free*
- *Faux foods labeled "low-fat" or "non-fat"*
- *Candy, gum, ice cream treats unless sugar–free or low "net-carb"*
- *Over-the-counter medicines and cough drops containing sugar, if there is a sugar-free alternative*
- *Spice mixes that contain MSG*
- *Worcestershire and soy sauces*
- *Hydrogenated fats, including margarine, shortening, and trans fat*

For now, all of these items will send you back to food cravings. When you get to a maintenance level, you will be able to enjoy some of the items on this list.

Foods to Stock

- *Calorie-free sweetener of your choice*
- *Liquid calorie-free sweetener*
- *Lemon and lime (fresh or juice)*
- *Meats and poultry without added broth*
- *Extra-virgin olive oil*
- *Sesame oil (unrefined)*
- *Fresh or frozen fish (uncoated)*
- *Fresh and frozen green vegetables (but not beans, peas or other legumes)*
- *Celery*
- *Lettuce, salad mixes, and spinach*
- *Avocados and olives (types of non-sugary fruits)*
- *Real heavy whipping cream*
- *Real butter*
- *Real cheese*
- *Real sour cream (not low-fat)*
- *Eggs (high in omega-3 fatty acids preferred)*
- *Nuts (without coating and not dry-roasted)*
- *100% pure baking cocoa*
- *Real mayonnaise*
- *MSG-free canned tuna packed in olive oil*
- *Pork rinds (unflavored, MSG-free)*
- *MSG-free sausage and bacon*
- *Sugar-free gelatin (Jello-O™) deserts*
- *MSG-free and sugar-free spice mixtures*

More information on food choice is in the chapter on shopping.

recipes and meal plan. More information about selecting the right foods is in the chapter on shopping.

When you look at the recommended foods, do not be alarmed if you see foods you do not usually eat. If there are foods to which you are allergic or will not eat for religious or other reasons, just skip them. If you find foods that you have never tried, be daring. This is a great time to break old habits.

In addition to food, there are a few items you will need to test yourself and monitor your weight loss. These are as follows:

- Glucose meter and supplies
- Bathroom scale
- Kitchen diet scale
- Multivitamins with minerals
- Sugar-free fiber supplement
- Ketone test strips
- "Calorie-counting" reference book

Each of these items has an important purpose, so do not skip this step. All diabetics should already be using their meter regularly, but if you are not, now is the time to get it out and check to be sure your supplies are fresh.

The bathroom scale is very important. Many dieters have learned to dread their scale, because of previous frustration with failed diets. Using this plan, you may learn to love your scale, because it helps you track steady progress. Watching your numbers go down can be rewarding.

Although you may already own a scale, see if yours can pass this test. First, can you measure small changes? A useful scale needs to be able to show you changes of half a pound or less. Bathroom scales that have small, unreadable dials or ones that round electronic readings to the nearest pound are not precise enough to be useful here. This diet works best when you get feedback on day-to-day changes. It takes a precise scale to do that. Your scale must also be reliable. Step on and off it a few times. If it gives you the same reading each time, it is reliable. If it does not, toss it in the trash before it does you more harm than good.

Surprisingly, a bathroom scale does not have to be perfectly accurate to work well. If your scale is precise and reliable, it does not matter if it gives you a number slightly different than a more accurate scale in your doctor's office. Just remember to track your weight on the *same* scale and under the same conditions, since you are interested in following the trend that the scale will show you.

You should also test your kitchen diet scale for precision and reliability, but it *does* need to be accurate. This will be the tool that lets you judge what size food portions work for you. There are good spring scales but an electronic scale can adjust to allow you to weigh food on a plate, making it easier to use. If you can not find a reasonable scale in a kitchen store, an electronic postage scale from an office supply store works just as well. Find a model with increments of less than an ounce.

A daily multivitamin supplement and mineral is essential for dieters, whether on this or any other diet. Individual needs and food choices will vary, putting dieters at risk of missing some important micronutrient. A daily multivitamin and mineral supplement is your best insurance against that occurring. Although there are claims made to the contrary, for this purpose almost any reliable brand will do.

Daily sugar-free fiber is an absolute necessity on this diet. Your body will process the food found in this diet with very little waste. That will result in little bulk for your bowel movements. Since your intestines have accommodated to larger amounts, the smaller amount of waste may just sit there until gradually, you become constipated. Adding fiber to your diet from the beginning prevents this problem. Do not wait until it happens. There are many fiber supplements at your pharmacy, but be sure they are sugar-free.

The oldest, most reliable supplement is psyllium fiber, in the form of Sugar-Free Metamucil™ powder. It requires you to stir a teaspoon into a glass of water and drink it quickly. Psyllium also comes in a capsule that is simpler to take, but the capsule may not have the same reliability. Some people prefer one of the newer types of tasteless fiber, such as *inulin,* that can be dissolved in your morning coffee or other beverage. Whichever you choose, follow the label directions and adjust the amount to fit your need so that the result is a daily bowel movement without straining or discomfort. The section on reading nutrition labels will tell you more about comparing these.

Ketone test strips may be familiar to anyone who has tried other low-carbohydrate diets. These come in a bottle of fifty and are usually found near diabetic testing supplies in the pharmacy. They are called *Ketostix™* or generically *Ketone Test Strips.* We will discuss how and why to use them shortly. While you are in the pharmacy, be sure that you have an adequate supply of fresh test strips for your glucose meter.

Many dieters already own a calorie-counting reference book of some sort. Most any one will do, if it shows grams of fat, protein, and carbohydrate for common produce, meats, and fish. Most of these books are thick from detailed and unnecessary listings of packaged products. The same information is always available on the package itself, where it will be up to date. You will need it for the fresh items that are not packaged. You may also be able to find that information on the Internet and skip the extra book.

This is enough preparation for most people. However, if you have had your gallbladder removed, or if your physician is concerned that you may develop gallbladder disease, pay close attention to the next few paragraphs. If you ever have difficulty digesting fat, consider using a product called MCT (*for Medium-Chain Triglyceride*) oil. MCT is a form of fat that is digestible without your body first breaking down the long chain of fat molecules that are normally strung together. It allows dietary fat energy to be used even for people who cannot easily digest fat. If you suffer from this difficulty, substitute MCT oil for other fats in the recipes found here.

Finding MCT oil may be difficult. Hospital pharmacies carry it, in an expensive pure grade. If a natural food store near you does not stock it in a consumer grade, you may be able to order it online or by phone. If you cannot find MCT oil, you may wish to try using unrefined coconut oil, available at specialty and natural food stores. It is a natural source of medium-chain triglycerides.

In addition, there is a medication that your doctor might prescribe called **ursodiol** *(or ursodeoxycholic acid),* which is prescribed as *Actigall*™ and under several other trade names. Research has shown it can prevent gallstone formation in many dieters. If you experience problems when eating fatty foods, talk to your doctor about starting that medication <u>before</u> you begin to diet. Additional information on special extras some people might need is in the chapter on supplements and special medications.

The chapter that follows will guide you through starting your diet by turning on your fat-burning switch.

Dieters and Gallbladder Disease

Your gallbladder is a small storage sac that holds bile produced by your liver. This supply of bile is then dumped into your intestine whenever it is needed to help break down long strings of fat before they are absorbed. Some people develop stones, inflammation, and even infections in their gallbladder. If your gallbladder has been surgically removed, you still produce bile but it can not be supplied in large quantities when needed.

Unfortunately, the following groups have a statistically higher risk of having gall bladder problems:

- *Women-especially those who have had children (the risk goes up with more children)*
- *People who are over 40*
- *People who are overweight*
- *People who are dieting*

Keep this in mind when dieting. If you find yourself unable to handle fat, developing symptoms such as fullness, nausea, bloating or diarrhea after eating fat, try changing to a different fat such as MCT oil and talk to your doctor about imaging studies to evaluate your gallbladder, as well as medication to dissolve stones and prevent their formation.

*If you develop abdominal pain, tenderness or discomfort, particularly in your right upper abdominal area under your rib cage, **seek medical help promptly**.*

Finding MCT oil

Suppliers and addresses can change,
so check
www.HippocraticDiet.com

for suggestions about obtaining MCT oil if
it is not available locally.

8

Starting to Diet

This plan has three phases, *starting, fat-burning* and *maintaining your weight.* This chapter is about starting, which is the shortest but trickiest part of this plan. Many people start this diet easily, but others may feel tired and irritable for a day or two. Diabetics have the extra task of holding all or most diabetic medication, while monitoring their sugar and keeping their physician informed. I advise my patients to start on a weekend or other time when they are not working, traveling, or scheduling important events.

The purpose of this starting phase is to rapidly move you off the "dietary cusp." A cusp is a sharp point, in this case at the intersection of sugar-burning and fat-burning. All weight-loss diets should have burning fat as their goal, but most diets keep you right at this intersection. Imagine yourself sitting on a sharp point. Keeping you at this point is very uncomfortable and makes many diets fail. When you are between sugar-burning and fat-burning, you can feel irritable, weak, confused, and you may be obsessing about food. *The starting phase of this diet is designed to get you past that point and into comfortable fat-burning as quickly as possible.*

The simplest way to tell your body to burn fat is through

total starvation or fasting. If you eat absolutely no food, your body makes the switch to burn its stored fat in a matter of days, but some people will have a difficult time with a total fast. This starting diet provides alternative strategies for those initial days. These strategies provide a partial fasting alternative and can be easier than observing a total fast.

If you were on medication and monitoring your glucose, what is its level the morning you start fasting and holding your medication? It should be no higher than on other mornings, before you began. Hopefully, it is normal or near normal, but many diabetics I see were nowhere near normal on their prior medication regimen. As the day progresses, your body should dump glycogen to keep your sugar level up. You should not be dropping too low, unless you still have medication on-board. If there is any question, call your doctor. Since you prepared a plan earlier, he or she should not be surprised by your questions. For some of my patients, I tell them that a reading in the high 100s is perfectly acceptable, but just for the day or two that they are in this transition. If they are higher, I will institute Metformin or increase the dose if already on it, provided that their diabetes has not already caused some kidney problems. Remember, this is not a do-it-yourself project. You must work with your physician on any medication changes.

As your stored carbohydrate glycogen is depleted, you will begin to transition to burning fat. Your glucose reading should fall to near normal levels. If it does not, keep your physician informed. Your diabetes may be moving closer to pancreatic insufficiency and you may need be treated similarly to a type 1 diabetic. Fortunately, the percentage of people who are at this stage is small. Even if you can not fully use this plan, close dietary monitoring will help you lose weight and control glucose, but you should <u>not</u> attempt coming off all medication.

The quickest strategy for starting is **calorie-free partial fasting** and the alternative is **fat-centered partial fasting**. Using either strategy, you deprive your body of sugar. That forces the hormones and neurotransmitters that regulate your hunger to cry out for sugar. Your body is then forced to burn its emergency supply of glycogen, the starch that provides a quick sugar fix. As you burn up that glycogen supply and sugar becomes scarce, your muscles begin burning fat, but your brain resists the change, and keeps using your remaining sugar. Your brain cells will wait while your sugar supply runs low. *Because of this, you may find yourself becoming anxious, grouchy or ill-tempered and have difficulty concentrating. **Schedule your personal events accordingly.** If you are an airline pilot or a brain surgeon, take a few days off!*

Once your change-over is complete, you will begin to feel re-energized. When your brain starts burning fat, subtle changes occur in your brain chemistry and neurotransmitter levels. As discussed earlier, fasting has been used to promote inner peace for thousands of years and in many cultures.

Getting High on Fat?

"Mary" attended a reunion after starting her diet. She worried that she would feel out-of-place, by not having alcohol. Instead, she reported that as she circulated, with club soda in hand, she felt wonderful. She said "I think the ketosis kept me mellow, feeling the high I would have felt having a drink, without touching alcohol."

Similar brain-chemistry changes may be the mechanism responsible for the benefits of a diet high in fish oil for mental health issues. This is an important breakthrough now being studied around the world .

Chapter 8   *Starting to Diet*

Once you have reached this fat-burning state, this plan is intended to safely keep you there. This is very different than remaining on that uncomfortable edge with other plans.

During this initiation phase, you may lose weight fast. This is sometimes called "water-loss" but is actually the result of glycogen loss. Glycogen weighs more than fat, so you lose weight faster when burning it off. In addition, glycogen is bound to water so the idea of water-loss is partially correct. This rapid loss of a few pounds is very important, but this is not the desired stage of steady fat loss. It is this rapid loss of weight that allows some diets to make claims about losing so many pounds in just a few days.

Exactly how long this transition to fat-burning takes will vary, because some people may have become physically addicted to high-carbohydrate foods. The important enzyme pathways that turn stored fat into burned-up energy may be weak. If skipping a meal puts you in a bad mood or keeps you from thinking clearly, you may have weakened pathways for burning fat. If so, allow yourself a little extra time for this starting phase.

Atrophy

If you were ever in a cast, you experienced atrophy. Your body is designed to "use it or lose it". As cells wear out, your body favors replacement of things that are active. When your cast came off, your weakened limb needed exercises or therapy to regain strength

Similarly, brain connections, neurotransmitter levels and enzyme pathways respond to use. You are trying to turn on switches to burn fat that are rusty and stiff. Be patient, your body's abilities will come back.

Diabetes Recovery

Your choices for calorie-free partial fasting are simple. During those few days, do not eat anything containing significant amounts of calories. Limit what you eat to the following list:

Things that You Can Have
During Your Calorie-Free Fast

- Water, coffee, tea and calorie-free diet soft drinks
- Artificial sweeteners
- Sugar-free chewing gum
- Celery
- Most spices (excluding MSG)
- Medicines prescribed by your physician
- Sugar-free vitamin and mineral supplements *(required)*
- Sugar-free fiber supplements *(required)*

You should drink plenty of water or other fluids during this time. Following this method should send your body into fat-burning as rapidly as a total fast, without feeling as deprived.

However, a calorie-free fast may be too severe for some. If you try this and find yourself ready to give up, switch to the plan for a fat-centered partial fast. You can add anything on this next list, provided that you do not exceed sixty to seventy grams of fat each day. Because these may contain some energy, including small amounts of protein and carbohydrate, this may stretch out your starting phase for another day.

Items on this next list are explained in the sections on recipes and shopping. Read those sections, so that you do not get the wrong product or use a recipe too high in the wrong ingredients.

Some Foods You Can Add to a Fat-Centered Partial Fast

- *Extra-virgin olive oil and unrefined sesame oil*
- *Real heavy whipping cream (not prepared whipped cream!)*
- *Real sour cream*
- *Real mayonnaise*
- *Real butter*
- *Real homemade cream soda*
- *Sugar-free Jell-O™ (in limited amounts)*
- *Real homemade whipped cream*

Use the sesame or olive oil, mayonnaise and the bleu cheese dip *(see the chapter on Meal Plans and Recipes)* on the celery. The homemade real whipped cream *(also in the recipes)* adds sparkle to your Jell-O.™ Use the cream in your coffee. Follow the recipe for real cream soda. *"Real"* is the key word in several of these. You may have become so accustomed to substitutes that the use of real ingredients instead of sugary counterfeit substitutes may seem strange. Follow the recipes closely until you learn the basics. Later, you are free to go ahead and develop your own variations. Although you will only be on the starting phase of this diet for a few days, continue to enjoy some of these treats throughout your diet.

You only need to stay in this starting phase briefly. Most people will take about two-to-three days. Once your body starts to naturally break down its stored fat, chemical changes in your blood will signal that you are ready to move on to the fat-burning phase of the diet and resume eating.

Diabetes Recovery

How will you know when you reach this stage? A few people may notice some difference in their urine and a fruity taste in their mouths, but the only reliable way to know when fat is coming from storage is a simple home test. You will have completed the starting phase when this test becomes positive.

You will now get to use ketone test strips that you purchased. To use a test strip hold it by the plastic end while dampening the paper end in your urine stream. Try to time it nearer the end of your urine stream. Ketones are fat and may float on the urine in your bladder, giving you an inaccurate low reading at the beginning of your urine stream. If you find this awkward, you may catch some urine in a disposable cup and dip the test stick. Either way, it takes just a drop to get it damp. Remove it and wait fifteen seconds, as directed by the instructions that come with it.

If you are burning enough stored fat to show in your urine, the indicator will change color. Compare the strip to the comparison chart on the side of the bottle, which resembles the picture below, although your chart will be in color. The colors will vary between a pale beige and a deep reddish-brown brick color.

Urine testing is never as accurate as blood testing, but it is painless, inexpensive, and done in the privacy of your home. For the purpose of monitoring your diet, this test is good enough.

Do not expect it to show much on the first day, but by the second, or third day the color should reach *moderate* or *large*. Once you reach that point, you are ready to move on and start following the suggested meal plans and recipes.

In the past, some diabetics were taught to fear ketosis. It is a danger sign for Type 1 diabetics when associated with very high sugar levels. It is <u>not</u> a danger sign for type 2 diabetics, when it is the result of deliberate dietary changes and associated with normal or near normal sugar levels.

Ketones are slightly acidic. Initially, when your body changes to fat-burning it will create an acidic condition in your blood called *acidosis*. Unlike the dangerous diabetic ketoacidosis coupled with high sugar levels found in poorly controlled Type 1 diabetics, this mild acidosis is within the range to which your body easily adjusts. Your body will rapidly neutralize this condition on its own.

If you or your physician want to speed up this adjustment process, drinking an occasional glass of water in which you have dissolved a teaspoon of bicarbonate *(baking soda)* may speed up the natural adjustment process.

Now, you can go back to eating meals. You will be surprised, for your appetite will be diminished and you will be content with the smaller portions outlined in this plan.

9

Eating to Recover

Now that you are in solid fat-burning, it is time to begin eating. You already may have lost a few pounds while you were getting started. Now, you will be able to eat a variety of foods in the right amounts and proportions. This balance should keep you from feeling deprived or hungry while you continue to lose weight at the rate of two or more pounds each week. The daily plan shown here is an example, with additional plans and recipes provided in a later chapter.

Some people prefer to be told exactly what to eat every day, while others prefer independence in their food selections. Consider the meal plans and recipes a starting point. In later chapters, you will see how simple it is to create new recipes or modify others to fit this diet. You may share your creations with others at www.HippocraticDiet.com. Some of the recipes given in here originated with dieters and diabetics like you.

I have found that most people who are successful like to start out by closely following recipes and meal plans for a few days. Once they see how easy and effective these are, they begin to experiment and change things. Keeping close watch on your own progress is the best way to see what changes really work well.

As you transition to the meal plan, monitor your glucose readings carefully. Use a daily diary, explained in Appendix C, to record readings and notice how certain foods cause them to change. Ideally, two hours after you have eaten, you should see readings return to a normal baseline. You may not be perfect, depending upon how far gone you were before you started this plan. As an example if in the past you were horribly out of control with an A1c of 10 and glucose readings two hours after eating of 200 despite medication, a slightly elevated

---

A Typical Day's Meal Plan

Breakfast
Coffee (or tea or chocolate)
made with real cream and non-calorie sweetener
Large egg, cooked your way
Strip of thick sliced bacon
(or msg-free sausage or fried smoked salmon)

Lunch
Non-calorie beverage
Green salad with extra-virgin olive oil based
dressing

Dinner
Non-calorie beverage
Small portion salmon fried in olive oil (or butter)
with spices
Asparagus dressed in real mayonnaise curry
dressing
Chocolate cream desert

Snack
Portion of nuts

---

reading of 130 taken 2 hours after eating and on no medication is tremendous progress and should be acceptable to your physician. In fact your physician should be ecstatic. On the other hand, if your diabetes was in an early stage, you should try for readings that are completely normal. With time, your body will undergo healing and demonstrate better control. Keep your personal physician informed of your progress and your readings as you go along.

This is the point that you will learn how much control you exert over your own disease. You'll notice how certain foods and portion sizes keep the numbers higher than you wish. This is why your log is so important. As you see how you can control this, you learn you are not a helpless victim. You are learning to use a powerful tool and being given immediate feedback. What is the point of close monitoring of your blood sugar, if you do not put what you learn to good use?

All the meal plans roughly follow the 60-40-10 plan. These are for a person who uses about 2,000 kilocalories or more of energy daily. Some people who are smaller, older, or less active may burn fewer calories and need to adjust their meal plan amounts downward.

The 60-40-10 daily plan	
Fat	*60 grams (but not more than 70)*
Protein	*40 grams (or up to 65 if carbohydrates are cut)*
Carbohydrate	*10 grams (or less if you want more protein)*

When you switch from the initiation phase to this phase of your plan, it could not be simpler. You will be pleasantly surprised at how you feel full, eating portions that are much smaller than you were used to in the past. Start by following the meal plans and recipes supplied in this book. Swap around those things you do or do not like but keep an open mind about recipes and foods you have not tried before. Continue to use the ketone test strips to be sure you stay at a moderate-to-high level of ketosis. Watch your scale and see if you can detect a quarter pound loss each day. See what works for you and adjust and personalize it to meet your needs.

As a diabetic following this plan, you have a significant advantage, provided you are making full use of your glucose meter. You can see the exact effect of particular food and portion size on your sugar readings.

This adds another dimension to your ability to personalize your diet to meet your needs. It is important from the very beginning. You should have an idea of what your glucose readings were in the past. Comparing these to what they are as you diet will give you a general idea of how much your diet is improving your control. In addition, if your diabetes has progressed to a more advanced stage, you can tell this, too.

How often you measure will depend upon your agreement with your physician. I believe that diabetic dieters will get the most out of this plan by checking their glucose levels four times each day. Do this in the morning, before eating as well as two hours after each meal. Use the diary explained in Appendix C to note the times of your meals as well as the times of your tests. As you do this, a clear picture will emerge of the relationship between these. You stop being the victim of a disease and instead will become the one in charge of your health.

Some people may noticed that too much protein at one time causes their sugar level to remain high hours after eating. They may find, as an example, that by paying close attention to portion size they can handle that item without problems. Others may notice that more than the smallest amounts of carbohydrate create difficulties but by adjusting their diet they can maintain a normal glucose levels.

These conditions are not always static. You are giving your body a vacation from the abuse of high glucose levels. This abuse caused impaired glucose tolerance, which worsened the situation. As the situation worsened, your pancreas became overtaxed and less able to respond with sufficient insulin.

By a taking a holiday from this abuse, some healing may take place. As time goes by, some damage will heal but you will be the first to detect this through close monitoring. Knowing how your body reacts to a particular foods, food combinations and portion sizes will allow you to take control of your disease and return to a normal but vigilant lifestyle.

How do you know what works for you? You will get to personalize your diet by tracking your progress, a skill you will learn using Appendix C.

Are You as Smart as Your Car?

Your car has a computer to vary the ignition timing and fuel injection between performance and economy modes. It can detect when you switch the octane level of your gasoline. Your body is infinitely smarter than your car. Right now, if it had your car's computer, it might be running in the trailer-towing mode.

After a few weeks you will get so used to your new diet that it will become second nature, but you should initially keep close track of your diet. The extra effort of jotting down a few notes daily can make the difference between you cruising along on your diet without difficulty or bumping up and down with plateaus and slow progress points.

All diets are infamous for plateaus, periods when the diet appears to not be as effective as when it first started. Many people think that they have reached a biologic "set point," although still overweight. That is another misconception that keeps people overweight.

Earlier, I mentioned the additional exercise workout you have been getting, just by dragging around that extra weight. As you diet, two things occur. One is that you start using energy pathways that are rusty and weak. They may not have gotten much use in years. As you diet, you are exercising those energy pathways and they begin to operate more efficiently. That will change your energy balance because your body realizes that you are in an energy deficit, and it is squeezing every last drop of energy out of the food you eat and your stored energy. As you lose fat, you are hauling less weight around, causing you to need less energy for the same routine daily activities. This makes you believe you have reached a set point, a weight you cannot go below. No, you have not. If you are still overweight and your energy needs have dropped, adjust your diet. *The 60-40-10 plan is a starting point.* Individualize it to your energy needs as they decrease.

The sample meal plans exist because people asked for more information when they were starting to diet. Rather than calculate what works for them, they were asking for a simple starting point. Some people continue to use them as a guide, but most dieters pick and choose the recipes and combinations they like after the first few weeks. Even using these starting recipes and meal plans, track them well. They are all approximations and cooking methods, even different brands of products or cuts of meat may alter them. The most useful adjustments to your diet will be those you develop yourself.

Some people were disappointed when I suggested keeping track of their diet because they had been unsuccessful in the past, having kept a food diary at sessions at a weight-loss chain or under direction of a hospital dietician. They had gone to that trouble and still had not been successful either controlling their diabetes or losing weight. When they found that they were doing both on this plan, tracking progress and adjusting their diet for good glucose control and weight loss made the extra effort worthwhile. Three months after beginning, when they saw the improvement in their A1c, it made it all worthwhile.

Every day of this plan offers new insight into what works and what does not. Food cravings that suddenly return can sabotage either your weight-loss or your maintenance. Many days a dieter brings the label from a suspicious food into our group meetings. More often than not, we find a triggering appetite stimulant cleverly hidden in the ingredients list. You will learn about avoiding those hidden things in the chapter on shopping. It is the one chapter I suggest you re-read periodically. There are so many ways the food companies can sabotage your diet that shopping will become a new experience.

When you complete your partial fast and begin to eat, you

will be happy to eat again but skeptical about the small portion sizes. Most of my dieters have been very surprised to learn that they were satisfied with these seemingly small portions. That is the magic of your body. The diet is not magic, but your body is. Despite years of abuse, it can return to knowing what is healthy and what it needs.

Those who are skeptical will try to cheat. They will reason that they can diet more slowly by not trying to create such a major change. They are wrong. Although they may lose a few pounds, they will be fighting constantly. Why? Because the conditions that signal your body to go into maximum fat burning with reduced hunger will be defeated by this cheating behavior. Instead of having an easier time, as they had assumed, they make it much harder. Instead of my lecturing them on their folly, I let the group teach them by example. When they see and hear how other members are rapidly losing weight by not taking shortcuts, they eventually change and the pounds begin to easily slide off for them, too.

Soon, I will explain how to track your progress and determine what works for you. Using the daily plans given here as a general diet is a great starting point for the average person, but who is that? Keeping a close watch on your daily progress and choices will make this plan customized and more effective for you.

You are not helpless in this fight for better health and this is not just a diet, it is a choice to follow a winning lifestyle. As you successfully diet, you will realize that you have regained control over this segment of your life, it can give you the confidence to take control of other, seemingly unrelated, areas of your life. The first choices you will make will be in the supermarket and in your home, as you learn how to fight the obesity epidemic for yourself and your loved ones.

Are you Suspicious?

You may have read about how, in the past, the tobacco company scientists manipulated cigarettes using additives that made their product more addictive.

In August 2005 the *Chicago Tribune* newspaper published a series of investigative articles. They revealed collaboration between tobacco company brain chemistry experts and food scientists working at a popular cookie company, which is owned by the tobacco giant.

Do you wonder what they discussed?

10

Foods to Avoid

Was Albert Einstein talking about you when he defined insanity as repeating errors of the past and expecting them to come out differently? For you, this means that you must be open to letting go of particular foods that are obesity traps. If you live alone, clean your cupboards. Give away or toss out any of the food discussed in this chapter. Set aside your feelings of what you paid for something. Do not use the excuse that a guest might ask for it.

If you live with others, this is a more complicated task. You may not wish to impose your food choices on others. You are taking control of your health, they are not. However, as they see you are serious about your diabetes recovery and weight-loss program, they will begin to see the results. Hopefully, they should be supportive and be willing to compromise.

Start out by cleaning out the most unhealthy foods that no one in your household should be eating. Keep the special foods you obtain for your plan separate from other family foods. Many dieters have learned that once they start cooking with real ingredients, their family wants to share these new dishes, but do not start out forcing your choices on others.

I have repeated a brief list of foods to avoid from the earlier

Chapter 10   Foods to Avoid

chapter on getting ready to begin. This chapter provides you more information about avoiding foods that may sabotage your weight-loss. Five important food selection rules to follow are the following:

1. *Avoid faux-foods*
2. *Avoid flavor enhancers*
3. *Avoid engineered fats*
4. *Avoid unnecessary carbohydrates*
5. *Read all labels suspiciously*

Avoiding faux-foods

Faux is the French word for fake. If you are buying inexpensive costume jewelry with fake stones, faux is good. In food, it is not. Pseudo-foods, even Frankenstein-foods, are some other terms that can be used to describe the unhealthy substitutes concocted by the food processing chemists. The opposite of faux is real. You may notice that I am avoiding the term "natural" to describe real foods. I do this simply because the food manufacturers have legally kidnapped that word, assigning it a new meaning that you will find hard to believe.

You are probably eating less real food and more faux-food than you imagine. What is the difference? Go to your kitchen cupboard or refrigerator. Read the ingredients list on any food you pick up randomly. Isn't it amazing? The question to ask yourself is "What are these ingredients and what do they do?" It is very likely that you do not know what half of them are or why they belong in this particular food. If that is the case, it is probably a faux-food. Please, do not blame the farmer. Farmers still supply real food but the profit is in the processing.

One example is the substitution of chemicals for real cream

Continued on page 102

Foods to Clear Out

- *Sugar, honey, corn syrup, maple syrup, and other sugary syrups*
- *Flour, corn meal, oatmeal, breakfast cereals and other grain products*
- *Potatoes, rice, peas, beans, spaghetti, noodles, pasta, and other starchy foods*
- *Bread, croutons, crackers, cookies, cakes, muffins, donuts, and other baked goods*
- *Soft drinks, except calorie-free products*
- *Alcoholic beverages*
- *Salad dressing containing carbohydrate or MSG (as most do)*
- *All fruit drinks and sugary fruits*
- *All soups, unless MSG-free (not "No added MSG)*
- *Dessert mixes, unless sugar-free*
- *Processed meats unless MSG-free*
- *Faux foods labeled "low-fat" or "non-fat"*
- *Candy, gum, ice cream treats unless sugar–free or low "net-carb"*
- *Over-the-counter medicines and cough drops containing sugar, if there is a sugar-free alternative*
- *Spice mixes that contain MSG*
- *Worcestershire and soy sauces*
- *Hydrogenated fats, including margarine, shortening, and trans fat*

For now, all of these items will send you back to food cravings. When you get to a maintenance level, you will be able to enjoy some of the items on this list.

Chapter 10   Foods to Avoid

Continued from page 100

in dairy products. Butterfat is the expensive part of the milk. Dairy farmers are paid for their milk based upon the amount of butterfat it contains. The remainder of the cow's milk is much less valuable. If the same amount of butterfat can be used to produce a pint of real sour cream or four pints of faux sour cream, which do you think brings the food processor more money?

The low-fat craze created a tremendous profit generator for food processors. The chemical companies that supply additives to the food processing companies are good at what they do. Good for them, bad for you. To see this difference, look in your supermarket dairy case for real sour cream. The ingredient list will list only one item, **cream.** Nothing needs to be added to a real product to make it taste like the real thing or look like the real thing or feel like the real thing. Now, look at the low-fat or non-fat sour cream sitting right next to it. It lists ingredients to artificially give it flavor, texture, and color. Take away the actual cream and you are left with a chemical soup.

Faux-foods are bad for you for many reasons. Typically, when a real ingredient is removed, unhealthy amounts of sugar are added. Many low-fat foods, which dieters think are lower in calories, often have enough sugar added to have far more calories than the real product. Of course, this extra sugar is especially bad for diabetics. Faux-foods contain a mixture of chemicals designed to fool you by attempting to imitate not only the flavor, but also the texture and color of the real product. The most notorious among these are the glutamate flavor-enhancers, substances that dieters must avoid.

When original, real fats are removed, they are often replaced by the cheapest vegetable oils, deliberately hydrogenated to physically resemble what they replaced and

---

Have You Ever Visited
Colonial Williamsburg, Virginia?

Homes in Colonial Williamsburg are decorated in lovely and unique soft pastel shades, which modern paint companies have tried to duplicate. When the original colonists separated the butterfat from milk, they used that butterfat to produce butter and cheese. They used the leftover product for whitewash or tinted it for paint. Today, dairy processors sell as this product as non-fat skim milk.

---

full of dangerous *trans*-fatty acids. Real foods are typically fresher, while faux foods may have a much longer shelf life than real food. *(Who ever heard of cardboard going stale?)* Achieving that long shelf-life often requires the addition of even more worrisome chemical preservatives.

Sometimes laws and regulations require faux-foods to use truthful names and sometimes they do not. Look for the word **"Real"** in the product name but always continue to read the ingredient label. "Real mayonnaise" by regulation, must contain eggs and oil in certain amounts, while other "light" mayonnaise and other imitation spreads do not contain the same amounts of these ingredients. Both real and imitation versions usually contain spices. Although flavor enhancers may exist in either version, they are more likely to be found in the imitation substitute. Similarly, real butter does not need artificial ingredients but margarine is always artificial. Still, you need to be aware that not all butters are the same. Butter usually contains cream and salt, yet some processors add flavor and texture enhancers, so once again, read the ingredient label carefully. With time and practice, you will learn which products are the purest, which brands sold in your region are real food and which are not. It is a sad commentary that it is not always possible to find pure products but try to avoid faux-foods and eat pure foods wherever possible.

I have been using words such as *"pure"* and *"real"* avoiding the use of the word *"natural."* Most people think they know what "natural food" means and may picture a small grocer selling only the purest organically grown products direct from a small local and family-owned farm. Unfortunately, the food-processing industry has stolen that meaning from us. If we go to the dictionary, we can find more than a dozen meanings listed for the word *"natural."* When we think of the word *"natural"* regarding food, we might think of the dictionary definition **"not altered or treated or disguised."** My dictionary even uses *"natural coloring"* as an example of that definition. It would seem common sense to use this definition, and, if so, consumers could have confidence that a natural product was the real thing.

Unfortunately, there is another dictionary definition—the one that the food industry regulators have chosen. That definition is **"present in or produced by nature."** Using that definition, **any product is *"natural"* if it is made from something that ever grew, moved, or crawled**, whether or not it has any relation to the food in question!

I must warn you, this is a true example which may make you nauseous. Products such as strawberry yogurt and strawberry ice cream may contain a red dye listed as "natural coloring." Many consumers would assume that a "natural" coloring for strawberry would come from strawberries.

However, in the strange world of legislation and regulation designed by the food-processing industry, this additive is as far from strawberry as you can imagine. The "natural" coloring used is often cochineal dye, a red dye made of the dried and pulverized bodies of female cochineal insects of the beetle family *Dactylopiidae*. The food companies could easily use a red dye made from other chemical substances, but if they did, they would be required to identify it as artificial coloring. Instead, to fool the health-conscious consumer who is trying to avoid additives, they use crushed, dried beetle juice!

There is a consumer movement to stop this misleading labeling for this one particular insect product. The pro-consumer group, Center for Science in the Public Interest (CSPI), had petitioned the U.S. Food and Drug Administration to require different labeling for this one particular additive. After many years of complaints, the FDA finally ruled in 2009, that beginning in 2011 food manufactures will have to name this dye on their labels. I doubt that many people will know that *"carmine"*, one of the allowable names, means an insect dye. Unfortunately, this small step does not address the larger issue. Changing the labeling for this particular item, still does nothing to restrict the continued misuse of the word *"natural"* on thousands of other items that are similarly misleading. **Protect yourself from faux-foods by never trusting the word *"natural"* on an ingredient list without a specific and clearly understandable explanation of what the so-called natural ingredient actually is, where it came from, and why it is present in that food product.**

Who Can You Trust?

It is tough to avoid faux-foods and unwanted ingredients. I once visited the retail shop of meat-packing plant in an Amish farm area. I was shocked when I read the list of ingredients for their *"Farm-Fresh Amish Country"* processed meat products. They contained the same preservatives and glutamate flavor-enhancers as any cheap supermarket product. Since then, I have learned that these small producers buy their ingredients pre-mixed and can not purchase additive-free spice mixtures.

Read every product label carefully !

Avoiding Flavor Enhancers.

When I suggest avoiding flavor-enhancers, do not think that flavor-enhancers are some sort of spice. Spices have a taste or a fragrance of their own, which may complement the taste of a food. Flavor enhancers have no inherent taste. Their role is to amplify whatever other flavors may be present, whether those flavors are real or artificial.

MSG, which stands for **monosodium glutamate** is the prototype of all the glutamate flavor enhancers that dieters must avoid. You may have heard about the controversy surrounding MSG for years; yet, many of my patients do not even understand why it is added to processed food. Some people wrongly believe that it is a preservative of some sort. It absolutely is not a preservative, but just the opposite. As a powerful flavor-enhancer, it was first used in Asian cooking not to preserve food but to make old, stale food taste fresh and flavorful.

Simply put, MSG works by turning up the volume in our taste buds. In much of Asia, food is never brought to the table with a knife. Instead, it is cut into bite-sized portions before cooking. If this is done too far in advance, the cut food loses its freshness and is less flavorful. Adding MSG makes the stale food taste fresher, by amplifying the flavors that remain.

I am told that MSG and related compounds rarely occur in nature, with the possible exception of these sources:

- Kombu, a Japanese seaweed condiment used as a flavoring.
- Fermented fish sauce, which has been used in some form in the West as a flavor-enhancer since ancient times.
- A rare form of bat found only in one small island of the South Pacific. Islanders consider it quite tasty but it has been suggested that it may be related to an unusual neurological disorder found on that island.

A Japanese chemist named Kikunae Ikeda invented synthetic MSG a century ago. He was curious as to why the seaweed condiment, Kombu, his wife cooked with always seemed to make her cooking tastier. After identifying the MSG compound, he found a way to synthetically produce it. Ikeda became wealthy, as MSG spread rapidly throughout Asia, largely because of the food freshness problem due to the Asian cooking style. It was eventually added to Japanese canned foods to make them taste fresher.

The rest of the world did not pay attention to MSG until after World War II. Americans returning from Asia had noticed how the Japanese canned products seemed to taste fresher and more flavorful than their American equivalents.

American food processors woke up to this supposed "miracle" of modern chemistry and began to add it to their products. Popular cookbooks advised young housewives to add a teaspoon of MSG to all their dishes. However, by the mid-1960s, warnings about MSG toxicity were beginning to be heard. Consumers became alarmed and MSG became a dirty word. Since then, the food industry has played a cat-and-mouse game with the public. The use of MSG in processed food continues unabated, but it is often disguised in such a way that the consumer is unaware of it.

The efforts of the food-processing industry to cloud the issue are reminiscent of earlier efforts when the tobacco industry was trying to pretend that tobacco was not harmful. Apologist scientists on the food-industry payroll continue to say that MSG is not harmful. They are better funded than those consumers, researchers, and physicians trying to spread the alarm. Public relations efforts include industry-bankrolled groups, which purport to represent consumers' food safety concerns but exist to claim that medical evidence condemning MSG is inconclusive.

About thirty years ago, the giant tobacco companies realized that fewer people were smoking and diversified to an industry that consumers could not avoid, buying control over food processing in the United States. Therefore, it should not be surprising to see similar tactics, which had worked for so many years with cigarettes.

All that being said, I am not going to go into detail about all of the alleged bad and dangerous side-effects of MSG. There are toxicologists and consumer advocates attempting to alert the public about those issues. I will let these other voices argue the toxic effects of this family of additives with the food industry. My reason for telling you, the dieting diabetic, to avoid MSG and similar flavor-enhancers is based upon the very same science that the food processors use to justify it. Simply put, MSG works magnificently as a flavor-enhancer and in doing so, it becomes a diet-buster and can worsen the diabetes epidemic.

When MSG is added to poor quality food or to an artificially flavored substitute for real food, it makes it taste much better. Try eating just one flavored chip or snack containing MSG. Just like they advertise, it really can be difficult to stop at just one. I am surprised that I have not come across cardboard with MSG added. The food-flavoring experts could probably make it quite tasty.

In fact, scientists in the 1960s first showed what a powerful diet-buster MSG was. Feeding similar food to two groups of animals, with only one group having MSG added, the MSG-eating animals ate more and ended up weighing more than their non-MSG counterparts. Food scientists have known about this research for forty years. More recent research paints a picture that is even worse. A group of German scientists took this research experiment one step further. After the MSG-fed animals had eaten more and gained weight, the scientist stopped adding MSG to their food, but that group continued to eat more and gain weight for months. That experiment illustrated how the effects of MSG-induced weight-gain continued and showed that the gain was not limited to the food to which MSG was added

Forgetting all the other alleged effects of MSG, this one issue should be enough to influence anyone needing either to

Chapter 10   Foods to Avoid

lose weight, control diabetes, or to protect his or her family. *The knowledge that it can make you eat more is reason enough to avoid MSG.*

Saying *"avoid MSG"* is easy but actually doing it is hard work. The reason that I labeled this section "avoid flavor enhancers" was that the food industry has gone to great lengths to hide MSG in many products. Although these flavor-enhancers all act the same way, the food industry has figured out many ways to fool the public into thinking that they are avoiding MSG. Our loose food regulations look at the letter of the law through the eyes of the food-additive industry while avoiding the intent of the law to protect the public.

Once consumers started attempting to avoid foods containing MSG in the 1960s, the food industry has been intent on finding *"clean"* alternatives. *"Clean,"* in this context, is industry terminology, which I have heard from food-additive representatives. *It does not mean free of MSG.* Instead, it means finding creative chemical ways to avoid having to say MSG on the label!

You need some explanation of how MSG works in your nervous system to understand how they can get away with this. Going back to the inventor, the chemist Ikeda had determined the chemical composition of MSG but had no idea why it worked. At that time, scientists recognized the four taste receptors (sweet, sour, bitter and salty) on the tongue. To explain the amazing result from MSG, Ikeda proposed the existence of an additional taste receptor variously called "umami" or " tasty."

The existence of nervous-system signaling chemicals or neurotransmitters was not known in Ikeda's time. Today, we know much more about monosodium glutamate. It is composed

110

of an atom of sodium (as found in table salt) attached to a molecule of glutamate, which is also known as glutamic acid. Glutamic acid is a common amino acid, one of the building blocks of protein throughout nature. You eat amino acids all the time, but, in nature, most are bound within the structure of the proteins we eat, whether that protein is from animal or vegetable sources.

Various normal cooking or processing methods may modify or break down miniscule amounts of protein, but, for the most part, amino acids are not separated and freed up until the protein we eat is broken down in the digestive process. MSG, on the other hand, hits our taste receptors as soon as the food containing it reaches our mouths. MSG can also pass directly into our bodies through the tissues of our mouth, skipping much of the process of digestion.

Glutamic acid is extremely important to our nervous system, because it serves as a neurotransmitter, a chemical that send messages from one nerve cell to another. Glutamate is found as a neurotransmitter sending signals between the nerve cells judging taste in our brain. These cells in our taste pathways can be falsely stimulated. This false stimulation of this important nervous system pathway is similar to the way that many other drugs work. Such false triggering of important brain pathways is how many types of addictive drugs work, even heroin and cocaine. Glutamic acid, when freed up from natural protein, can be used as such a drug. Attaching it to an atom of sodium allows it to easily reach the nervous system pathways that tell us how much flavor a food contains. **It chemically turns up the volume of any taste that is actually present, making it taste more flavorful and creating a desire to eat more.**

Chapter 10   Foods to Avoid

Some food-industry funded scientists and food-writers focused on Ikeda's old idea of a finding a *"tasty" or "umami"* receptor within the nervous system. The food industry hopes that this idea will deflect attention from the drug-like effect of MSG and other additives. Publicizing scientific debate about where in the nervous system MSG works attempts to avoid the discussion of the devastating impact that it has had. This is just like the earlier discovery of other neurotransmitter effects. In the 1970s, brain scientists discovered that the receptor sites for the natural endorphins in our brain were the same sites hijacked by opium and heroin. This important scientific knowledge did not make heroin addiction and its devastating consequences any more normal.

Whether MSG works at specific *"umami"* receptor sites or simply turns up the volume by overwhelming all glutamic acid pathways does not change the harm that it does by causing you to overeat. There are other scientists, not employed by the food industry, more worried about the toxic consequences of MSG. Those scientists point to evidence that MSG may over-stimulate the glutamate-dependent nerve cells in our taste pathways. This idea, called the *excitotoxin hypothesis,* claims that such overloaded cells may suffer long-term damage, which has lasting effects, as in the laboratory animals that just kept eating.

Yet, for the purpose of dieting, none of this matters. Your issue is that MSG is the prototype for many flavor-enhancing additives that influence how much you eat. As the food industry has added chemicals to more and more products, you become the victim. Again, I advise you to **avoid MSG because it is a diet-buster**.

It is not easy avoiding MSG because government labeling

Honest Labeling is Consumer Protection.

The first national Pure Food and Drug Act became law in 1906, when Teddy Roosevelt was President. One provision mandated honest labeling. At that time, millions of American women had become addicted to various "tonics" sold for "female complaints." These tonics temporarily relieved their symptoms but were impossible to stop taking. They often contained highly addictive combinations of opium, cocaine, and alcohol, but the user had no idea of their contents. This law preceded strict drug control, but it was highly effective in stopping the epidemic.

Once women realized what was in these potions, they stopped becoming victims. As sales plummeted, manufacturers had to change their formulas or go out of business.

---

regulations favor the synthetic food processors. Simply put, they allow food manufacturers to camouflage MSG. Although some products tell you they contain MSG *(provided you read the fine print in their ingredients list),* others go to great lengths to fool you. This *"clean labeling"* game has been going on for three decades.

MSG can be manufactured from a variety of processes. They all involve some method of breaking down a protein, whether animal or vegetable. As an example, you can ferment a broth of crushed vegetable, fish, or beef protein and let microbes break apart the protein into its various amino acids. Another way to create MSG is to use a solution that is heavily salted and let the osmotic pressure from the heavily salted water cause hydrolysis. This means a breaking apart, which frees the amino acids, letting them combine with salt solution.

Chapter 10   Foods to Avoid

These are over-simplified explanations of some complex methods devised by the food processing and flavoring industries over many years. They help explain why food labeling regulations give the food processing industry tremendous latitude. If the food processor adds powder from a large chemical drum labeled MSG, they must say MSG on the label of their finished product. However, if they add the chemical brew from a tanker car filled with one of the broth products I just described, they might be able to label their product as containing something other than MSG, such as:

- hydrolyzed vegetable protein
- HVP
- hydrolyzed soy protein
- hydrolyzed corn protein
- vegetable broth
- vegetable protein
- yeast extract
- fermented soy product

Those are just a few of the many aliases that MSG can take. More MSG aliases are listed in Chart 10-1 at the end of this chapter. Each of these products contains MSG or a similar chemical. Some names sound incomprehensible while others sound perfectly innocent. Vegetable broth sounds like some hearty dish that your grandmother might cook. Of course, you might wonder what grandma's vegetable broth was doing in your can of cheap tuna fish!

Another problem with MSG is the dietary "salt" issue. We have been told for several decades that everyone should cut back on their use of salt. This is a misunderstanding. The recommendation is actually for **sodium**, part of ordinary salt.

MSG is a source of sodium in processed foods, but the food companies obscure this by talking about salt.

Actually, even sodium reduction advice may not be for everyone. Many people with kidney, heart, and blood pressure issues must stay on sodium-restricted diets. Whether this is good advice for everyone else is questionable, and some other people may get too little sodium.

The vast majority of Americans do get a large amount of sodium in their diets. The press and the government say "salt," since chemically table salt is sodium chloride. However, salt is not the issue. It is the sodium portion that is. Often, people on such low-sodium diets are given potassium chloride, a healthier chemical form of salt, often called a salt substitute. Why is this important? Stop and think for a moment. Doctors and biologists understand that **sodium** is the issue, not "salt." Sodium is added to the food supply in any food containing *mono**sodium** glutamate.* If you are someone who has been told to reduce your "salt," try reducing your MSG.

These are just a few of the ways MSG can be hidden. This will continue to be a problem until there are adequate laws warning consumers about hidden or disguised additives. Look for foods that are clearly labeled as **"MSG-free"** or **"No MSG,"** but even then, read the label. Food companies continue to test their limits with the lax enforcement of labeling standards. Sometimes, they even advertise that they have not added MSG to their product, when in fact, they have added it in the form of "hydrolyzed vegetable protein" or "yeast extract." Never trust the phrase *"No Added MSG,"* it is as misleading as *"No Added Sugar."*

Do not be surprised at the many places you find MSG hiding. It is common in snack foods such as chips and coated nuts. It shows up in canned ravioli, seasoned french fries, frozen dinners, and in canned tuna fish. It is common in many restaurants and is sometimes found in the *"seasoned salts"* served at restaurants and perhaps found on your spice rack. After you begin to read labels closely, you should suspect it everywhere!

Avoiding Engineered Fats

Dietary fat has been given a bad reputation that it does not deserve. The type of fat you eat is more important than how much fat you eat. All people need fat in their diet, because although your body can create storage fat from extra energy, you need a few types of fats, called "essential fatty acids." These can only come from what you eat. On this plan, keeping the right proportion and amount of fat in your diet is an absolute necessity, because it is the trigger to burn up your stored fat. At the same time, it makes sense to distinguish good from bad fats, while you are changing your habits and lifestyle of many years.

Food scientists have used selective breeding, genetic engineering, chemical modification, and other methods to create substitutes for the healthiest fats. Try to avoid all of these engineered substitutes. Natural fats such as olive oil have been keeping people healthy since biblical times.

Later, we will discuss picking the very best fats, including those high in omega-3 fatty acids, such as those found in certain fish and those very high in monounsaturated fat, such as olive oil. Many people believe that all saturated fat is bad, but that is not the case. A diet with a reasonable amount of natural saturated fat found in dairy, meat, and poultry is perfectly healthy.

What are the unhealthiest fats? They are the artificially modified vegetable fats called *hydrogenated* or *trans*-fats. About a century ago, chemists discovered that if they took some of the very cheapest vegetable oils and chemically modified them through a process known as *hydrogenation,* they could thicken them and change their appearance and cooking characteristics. One of the first uses for these hydrogenated fats was in the baking industry. Hydrogenated fats were cheap and easy to use as substitutes for the butter or lard typically used as shortening in fine pastry.

Another use was for margarine, but initially, the public was not easily fooled by this cheap substitute. The typical margarine is made from an inexpensive vegetable oil, which has been synthetically hardened by hydrogenation. Hydrogenated fat produces a grayish-white substance that had no resemblance to butter. Dye is added to produce a butter-like color. Food shortages in both World War I and II created a temporary market for this inferior product, but people understood that it was a cheap substitute for the real product, butter.

Some states, particularly those with dairy industries, put legal restrictions on the sale and use of margarine. These restrictions were aimed at protecting the public from being sold these products without their knowledge. Today, these restrictions are all gone. Misinterpretation of scientific data beginning in the 1950s and 1960s led the public to believe that margarine was healthier than butter, since it was made from vegetable oil. The industry conveniently forgot to tell the public that once vegetable oil had been hydrogenated, it not only resembled saturated fat but did so in an unnatural and unhealthy way.

Canned vegetable shortening was sold to homemakers and began to replace butter and lard for frying and home baking. Industry *"partially hydrogenated"* liquid vegetable oils because hydrogenation also slows the rate at which oils turn rancid. This was important to the fast-food industry, since they typically keep large amounts of oil in open fryers for many days.

The public is just beginning to understand what chemists and physicians have known for a century. This hydrogenation process bonds together molecules in an unnatural way. These bonds face in the opposite direction of natural fats. They are called *trans*-fats, from the Latin word for "across." This is because the bonds holding these fat chains together cut across in this opposite direction. Unfortunately, our bodies do not deal well with this excess of backward-facing fat. As these fats are broken down, these oddly-bonded fragments end up creating health problems.

These hydrogenated or *trans*-fats are the real villains. People have been eating healthy natural fat for millennia. It is only in the last century that our food supply has been modified with this cheap substitute. **Never eat any food with the word *hydrogenated* in the ingredients list!**

Another unusual type of ingredient is sometimes called tropical oil, or may it be listed as vegetable oil, palm-kernel oil, or coconut oil. These oils, grown on a plantation in tropical climates, have an unusual characteristic, for although they are vegetable in origin, they contain a high degree of saturated fat, like meat and butterfat. Typically, they are then hydrogenated and used in cheap commercial baked goods. Again, always stay away from hydrogenated oil. In general, there is little good to be said for palm-kernel oil, but coconut oil has a special characteristic that some people may need. We discussed this earlier with the information about MCT oils.

What about fats that have been modified in other ways? That is a tough call. Today, plant scientists and genetic engineers are trying to manipulate vegetable oils that have been around forever. They are doing so to try to get these cheap vegetable oils to resemble some of the healthiest oils. This is a noble goal, but is it a good choice for you? The jury is still out on these manipulations of the food chain. If you can afford the admittedly high price of real olive oil, do you want to save a few pennies by buying a cheaper vegetable oil that has been manipulated to be "almost as good as olive oil"?

Going Sugar-Free

Going sugar-free is one of the healthiest things you can do, no matter what type of diet you follow. Sugar should be eaten only in context, that is, in the way sugar is found in nature. Do not be fooled by the "natural" label used to peddle certain over-priced fruit sugars to diabetics. Once in your body, sugars are converted to the common currency of *glucose,* no matter what their source.

For thousands of years, purified sugar was a relative rarity. It was considered a luxury. The main source of pure sugar was wild honey. Foods that were naturally high in sugar were not year-around foods. Typically, high-sugar foods such as fruit could be eaten only during a brief season. Otherwise, they would have to be preserved by drying, such as turning grapes into raisins, or they would naturally ferment to alcohol or vinegar.

Chapter 10   Foods to Avoid

Sugar extraction was developed in India more than two thousand years ago, but the process was a guarded secret, which spread very slowly to the rest of the world. Sugar was considered a rare spice and consumed in small quantities by the rich or royalty. Even then, doctors noted diseases associated with the beginning of sugar consumption.

The greatest change in human sugar consumption came about with the European colonization of tropical regions. The European nations used slave labor to mass produce sugar cane, turning a rarity into a cheap product. Human consumption of sugar has been growing steadily since that time. Beet sugar and corn syrup have been developed as even cheaper substitute sources of sugar.

Today, the developing countries are getting hooked on high-sugar soft drinks and sweets. Indeed, the growth of sugar consumption in the newly industrialized world has led to an epidemic of both obesity and diabetes in countries such as India and China, nations where we still picture starvation and malnutrition. Ironically, they are now plagued by both obesity and malnutrition, not in the same people, but side-by-side, as they move from poor agricultural economies to Western-style manufacturing economies!

In both people and animals, such sugar use is unnatural. This heavy year-around use of sugar is addictive, because in addition to tasting good, this over-use of sugar has set up bodily changes so that you constantly want to maintain a high-carbohydrate consumption level.. One of the most difficult issues in reducing sugar consumption is the acquired taste that the human race has developed in the past several hundred years. As you diet, your taste for sweets will diminish. As long as you keep away from the sugar rush, your taste for sweets will gradually change. In the meantime, use sugar substitutes. This will separate the taste craving that you have long associated with the sugar rush.

This means avoiding all food to which sugar has been added. This seems tough, until you have been weaned from the linkage between the sugar taste and the sugar rush.

Fortunately, there are many acceptable sugar substitutes. A debate has gone on for decades regarding potential health risks of sugar substitutes. More will be said on sugar substitutes in the next chapter. Remember, the debate about supposed harm from sugar substitutes is largely hypothetical, but the health risk from sugar is both real and devastating. **Do not be afraid of sugar substitutes, be very afraid of sugar.**

Many foods contain hidden sugar. Avoid all foods that claim that they contain half the sugar or light sugar. They are simply stating that they use less sugar than a worse product, often by combining artificial sweetener with real sugar. Always read the nutritional label to be sure that zero calories are listed under sugar.

The Food and Drug Administration requires that ingredients listed on the label should be in order of quantity. That means that if the greatest proportion of ingredients is sugar that should come first on the label.

Faux-food manufacturers have developed a clever way to trick the public and get around this requirement. By using two or three different types of sugar, although the total would be first on a label, the individual sugars are not listed first; they are hidden down in the list of ingredients. Another trick is to use chemical names for common sugars, hoping that you, the consumer, will not recognize this. Such names include sucrose, dextrose, lactose, glucose, fructose and many other chemical names ending in "ose." *Treat every "ose" name as just another sugar.*

Another food industry trick is to use concentrates that make pure sugar sound like a healthy natural food. Examples are corn syrup and fruit juice concentrate. We think of fruit juice as natural and healthy, so the food companies use this ploy to stuff children's drinks with inexpensive apple-juice concentrate from China. They then have the nerve to say *"no added sugar"* boldly on the label!

Corn syrup is a another cheap source of very pure sugar and modified corn syrup is a substance that has been changed to make it taste even sweeter. More than one food company lists *"refined cane extract"* as an ingredient on their label. Translated into plain English, *"refined cane extract"* is actually ordinary table sugar!

As you have been reading this chapter, you may have been feeling that points I have been making were exaggerated. I would not blame you, for many of my patients have wondered this until their next trip to the grocery. Once they begin to read labels closely, they are amazed at what went into the supposedly healthy food that they thought they had been purchasing. Now, they are all devoted and somewhat paranoid label-readers.

Read all food labels suspiciously!

Chart 10-1

Many Names of Hidden Glutamate Flavor Enhancers

Certainly or Probably Contains MSG

Autolyzed "anything"
Autolyzed plant protein
Autolyzed yeast
Calcium caseinate
Disodium inosinate
Disodium guanylate
DSG
DSI
Glutamate
Glutamic acid
HPP
HVP
Hydrolyzed "anything"
Hydrolyzed corn protein
Hydrolyzed soy protein
Hydrolyzed plant protein
Hydrolyzed vegetable protein
Monopotassium glutamate
Monosodium glutamate
Sodium caseinate
Textured protein
Vegetable broth
Yeast extract

Often Associated with MSG Containing Foods

Annatto
Barley malt
Broth, stock or bouillon
Caramel flavoring or coloring
Carrageenan
Citric acid (when processed from corn)
Corn syrup and corn syrup solids
Cornstarch
Dough conditioners
Fermented "anything"
Flavors, flavoring, seasonings, spice, extract, reaction flavors
Flowing agents
Gelatin (except gelatin desserts)
Gums
Lipolyzed butter fat
"Low" or "No-fat" items
Malted barley
Maltodextrin
Modified "anything"
Modified food starch
Natural chicken, beef, or pork flavoring
Pectin enzymes
Protease
Protease enzymes
Protein-fortified milk, whey-protein, whey, milk powder, dry milk solids, whey protein isolate or concentrate
Protein-fortified "anything"
Rice syrup
Soy, wheat, rice, or oat protein
Soy sauce or extract
Soy-protein isolate or concentrate
Ultra-pasteurized "anything"

or
Any Ingredients that Appear Out of Place for the Food They Are In

11

Going Shopping

The key to this diet being effective is being very aware of what you eat. The simpler and healthier the ingredients you use, the better off you are. Allow more time for your shopping. As you begin to scrutinize the food you purchase, you will find that reading labels takes time. Gradually, as you discover what items to trust and what to avoid, your shopping trips will return to normal. Until then, keep reminding yourself to read both the ingredients list and the nutritional labeling to discover what you are really eating. Here are a number of simple rules to help you:

- *Avoid all sugars*
- *Fresher is always better*
- *Ignore phony health claims*
- *Do not trust the word "natural" without proof*
- *Avoid ingredients you do not understand*
- *Pick the product with the shortest ingredient list*
- *Do not be afraid to spend a little more for better foods*
- *Learn what foods you enjoy on this diet and use them*

Chapter 11   Going Shopping

There are some federal regulations about how food processing companies have to structure their labels. Although they try to be "creative," they have to adhere to a certain style in these labels. It is important that you learn how to read this important information. You may know some of these conventions but others may be a revelation to you.

There is almost always an ingredients list. The exception is for some products with only a single ingredient. As an example, a spice labeled "*black pepper*" might not have an ingredients list but a spice labeled "*seasoned pepper*," which contains multiple ingredients would need an ingredients list. All ingredients are listed in order of quantity. Therefore, the first ingredient on the list is present in the largest quantity while the last ingredient is there in the smallest quantity.

Many consumers already know this. Some shoppers who want to avoid high sugar foods try not to buy foods where sugar is listed as the first ingredient. Food companies know this and deliberately avoid placing sugar first on the label, particularly for children's items. As we discussed previously, the way that they do this is devious but perfectly legal. Instead of using one type of sugar, they may mix two, three, even four separate types of sugar. This brings the percentage of each type down so that another ingredient takes first place on the label.

Look for short ingredient lists. Generally, the purer the food, the fewer the number of ingredients, so longer lists often spell trouble. Look for any of the hidden or suspicious forms for MSG. Be suspicious of ingredients you do not recognize. One dieter recently told me "since starting this diet, I do not buy any food with ingredients that I cannot pronounce." That is some pretty sound advice. Although it may make you avoid some foods with innocent ingredients, it will prevent many mistakes.

Do not forget that the government allows many different names for the same ingredient. This freedom allows ridiculous attempts to fool the consumer. An example is one product where the first ingredient listed is *"evaporated cane juice."* Juice sounds healthy, does it not? If you pause a moment to think, you will realize the *"cane"* is sugar cane. *That means evaporated cane juice is just plain old sugar.*

Do not be content just because you recognize the names of everything. Pause a moment and question why an ingredient is there. Words like gelatin or broth can be innocent enough in the right context or they can be deceptive ways of describing ingredients you wish to avoid. Be suspicious when you notice something that does not seem to belong. Be suspicious of the word natural, as in *"natural flavoring"* or *"natural coloring."* Do not forget that the FDA considers creepy-crawlies to be natural, as in allowing crushed red beetle juice to be called *"natural coloring"* for strawberry yogurt!

Some people advise "shopping around the perimeter of the supermarkets" to find the purer foods. There is truth to this advice, but it is often not sufficient. What they mean by shopping around the perimeter is to totally avoid all the processed foods. The perimeter or wall of a typical supermarket often contains the produce department, the dairy case, and the meat and fish departments. Unfortunately, the dairy case also contains artificial creamers, dairy products altered with faux ingredients, and similar items. The meat department may contain meat and poultry injected with flavor-enhancing broth. The fish department may contain frozen pre-seasoned fish loaded with MSG.

Despite all this negative advice, you will quickly become

quite positive about shopping. Once you know how to determine what is good and bad for your diet, you will no longer have to read dozens of labels in the store. Just be prepared for a long visit the first time or two that you go to the supermarket.

This is an example of an actual "Nutrition Facts" box followed by an explanation of how to use it. Next to the ingredients list, this is the second most important piece of information on any packaged food. Read the explanation to learn about the key areas pointed to by the numbered arrows.

Diabetes Recovery

1. The box is headed by the words "Nutrition Facts" in large bold print. Most products contain this box. The only exception is for a product in a very small package such as candy or gum. If there is not enough room to use the box format, the manufactures will sometimes provide the same information in a textual format, usually in extremely fine print.

2. The next line explains the serving size. In this case, it is an individual fish fillet weighing approximately six ounces.

3. The next line tells you how many servings are in this package. In this case, there are six frozen fish fillets in one container. Be careful here. There are some items that are sold as individual portions; yet, the label says that the container has multiple portions. One notorious example is individual vending machine bottles of cola that are clearly sold for individual use; yet, the label shows multiple servings. This enables the manufacturer to imply lower calorie counts per serving than is actually the case.

4. Total fat is the first major category. In this case, the serving of fish contains twelve grams of total fat. The subheadings showing the type of fat are sometimes useful in understanding more about the food item, but they are often incomplete. Ignore the column labeled percentage daily value.

5. The next item of importance to you is total carbohydrate. In this case, the fish contains no carbohydrates, which is generally good for this diet. There may be additional subheadings under this category, which we will explain shortly.

6. Protein is the next significant item. In this case, the fish contains forty-one grams of protein in this single filet.

If you were considering this for dinner, note one slight

problem. You remember the 60-40-10 suggestions? This single fish fillet contains your entire day's worth of protein. Unless you were only having one meal that day, this would not be a wise choice. The solution is simple. Go back to the serving size and halve it, so that you only have three ounces of fish. Then it becomes an entirely appropriate portion.

When reading these charts, be watchful, for there may be hidden items. For example, a product's ingredients list may show that it contains sugar yet the "Nutrition Facts" may state that it contains zero grams of sugar and zero calories from sugar. What is happening? The government regulations allow the manufacturer to round down, so a product with less than one gram of sugar might say zero, while it actually contains a small amount. This may or may not be important to you, depending on how much you actually plan to use. If the ingredients list says it contains sugar, take it into account and add a small amount in your calculations.

Keep in mind that anything outside the ingredients list and Nutrition Facts box is subject to a different set of rules. Lawyers and advertisers use the term *"puffery."* Legally, puffery refers to fanciful statements that are made to make a product sound good. They are often exaggerated facts or "puffed up" features about a product. The only time the government regulators step in is when they decide these statements are harmful.

Often, a competitor will make a complaint to the government, feeling that exaggerated claims give its competitor an unfair advantage in the marketplace. One example might be a food product that claimed it could prevent cancer. A competitor could complain and government regulators could rule that making such a health claim was wrong. On the other hand, if the government became convinced that the food manufacturers had done nothing wrong and allowed them to continue, their competitor would feel that they had to make similar claims to maintain their share of the market. Although such claims may seem outlandish, they may be half-truths. Claims like this are not as tough to make as claims made on a new medicine.

A pharmaceutical manufacturer claiming that a drug might treat or prevent cancer would have to spend hundreds of millions of dollars testing and proving this to the satisfaction of government regulators. On the other hand, an advertising department that learned that one ingredient in a particular food might help in some health problem has a far lower standard to meet. Many products appear on the market with puffery on the front of label that imply they will make you healthier, thinner, prettier, and smarter. Treat those claims for what they are.

An oddity about food labels is that they must contain information about nutrients that your body will not use. As an example, fiber that is not digestible by people is still chemically a carbohydrate. The government regulations require that these carbohydrates be included in the total carbohydrates shown. However, they can then be shown under the subheading of "Fiber" and you are supposed to know enough to subtract this. Perhaps the expert genius who thought this up was mixing up people with cows, since cows are able to digest this fiber.

Another subtraction should be done for "*sugar alcohols,*" the chemical name for a group of substances that are neither what you would commonly think of as either sugar or alcohol. Instead, these are chemicals that should be treated as artificial sweeteners, but with a peculiar twist. They resemble sugar in the molecular region that matches our taste buds, so that you taste them as sugar but they do not match closely enough for your digestive system to use. If you see the term "sugar alcohol" in the Nutrition Facts box, once again, you subtract. You may also recognize them in the ingredients list, if you see a name ending in the letters *"ol,"* such as *"sorbitol."*

Here is an example of what you must do when seeing either sugar alcohol or fiber listed in the carbohydrate section. This example is from a label for a sugar-free candy.

Nutrition Facts

Serving Size 3 pieces (43g)
Serving Per Container about 2

Total Fat 12 g

Total Carbohydrate 24 g
  Dietary Fiber 2g
  Sugars 0g
  Sugar Alcohol 22 g

Protein 2g

In this case, you may subtract both the fiber (2 grams) and sugar alcohol (22 grams) from the total, resulting in 0 grams net carbohydrate! The same regulations that prevent the manufacturer from showing this accurately in the "Nutrition Facts" box do allow the company to brag about it on the front of the package. Depending upon whether they are marketing to diabetics, dieters, or to others, they <u>may</u> chose to advertise this as "Net Carbs" on the front of the package. You will find these sorts of statements on <u>some</u> lines of diet candy and ice cream, but there is little consistency.

Before you get too excited at the thought of candy and ice cream that you may eat on this diet, there is a down-side. Bacteria digest sugar alcohol. All those sugar-alcohol carbohydrates that your body cannot digest end up in your large intestine, where your normal intestinal bacteria feast on them. As a result, if you have more than a little, you may get gas and diarrhea as you overdo these sugar-free treats. People seem to differ in how much they can tolerate, so please be careful. Just because the package says a serving is three pieces, you do not have to follow that. Additionally, some diabetics do see an increase when they take their meter reading after eating these products. That implies that as these sugar alcohols break down, some portion may be absorbed. If you try a product like this, start with just one.

Now, begin your trip through your local supermarket. Walk in the door and turn right toward produce. The fresh fruits will have to wait until you level off at your maintenance phase. Instead, head for the vegetables. Stock up on lettuce in any variety you like. You may want fresh spinach for salad or cooking. Prepackaged lettuce mixtures are fine, provided they do not include any flavorings or dressings. You may want some celery for dips. Red and green peppers are a good choice to add some flavor to your cooking. Broccoli and asparagus are more good choices in the vegetable section. Cauliflower will be very useful to you, even if you do not eat it now, because it is found in some recipes as a potato substitute. You may be skeptical about that but once you have tried the recipes, you will understand why people often prefer it. If you like coleslaw, shredded cabbage is okay in moderation, but do not use it for a large vegetable course. Skip the starchy foods, such as beans, potatoes and beets.

If there is an olive bar in the vegetable department and you like olives, they are a welcome addition to this diet. Canned olives are good, too. The Manzanilla variety of olives are high in healthy olive oil.

Tomatoes are high in carbohydrates, so use them sparingly. Purchasing grape tomatoes is one way to control the amount you eat, since you can just use one or two as a flavoring on your salad. Onions contain carbohydrates, so if you use them in cooking, limit yourself to small amounts for flavoring. Try to avoid caramelizing them in cooking, as that turns their starch into sugar. Carrots are carbohydrate-containing root vegetables, so do not buy regular-size carrots. If you want to use them as a dip or a garnish, get those small, pre-peeled baby carrots and use them in moderation.

Next, move to the section where salad dressings and toppings are sold. If you use a bacon-like topping on your salad, switch to the real thing and be sure it is MSG-free. Salad dressings are going to be much tougher. You will be very disappointed as you read the ingredients list, because most of the bottled salad dressings contain MSG, sugar, or both. The powdered salad dressing spice mixtures that you mix with your own oil and vinegar are usually no better than the bottled products.

Salad dressings should be essentially free of carbohydrate so read the Nutrition Facts box. If your market has a section containing refrigerated salad dressings, you may have better luck. You will probably end up using some of the homemade salad dressings from the recipes we have given you or using simple oil and vinegar on your salads.

This is a good time to stop and buy vinegar. Ordinary white vinegar is nutrient free, while other vinegars, such as wine, malt or cider vinegar may contain traces of carbohydrate. Avoid balsamic vinegar, since it is made by mixing wine vinegar with *grape must*, a form of concentrated grape juice which adds a significant amount of carbohydrate.

Next, move on to the oil section. As you have probably already guessed, I am going to suggest that you stock up on extra-virgin olive oil. It is the best all-around type of oil that you can use. If you do a significant amount of deep-frying you probably already have some peanut oil. It is fine for this purpose. If your market carries it, pick up some unrefined sesame oil to try on your salads. You may have to look in the gourmet foods department or go to a health food store to find this product. Try to avoid soybean oil, cotton seed oil, and anything generically labeled "vegetable oil." Avoid all products labeled "shortening."

Find the spice aisle. Here you can experiment with a variety of spices that you may not have tried before. Virtually all pure spices are fine on this diet. Spice mixtures require more caution so read all of the ingredients list. Many mixtures contain MSG and some contain sugar. There are some excellent mixtures that will add a spirit to your cooking without any MSG or sugar. You will be amazed at the way real spices can bring out the flavor of real food without artificial flavor enhancers. Some recipes in this book call for items popular in Latin America, such as chipotle sauce and other spices. Many markets today have a separate ethnic food section where you can find these.

If you are near the condiment section, look for a real

mayonnaise in a brand that you like. *Real mayonnaise* is one of those regulated names and must contain proper amounts of oil and eggs. Beyond that, it may contain a lot of other unnecessary ingredients. Check the ingredients and go for the shorter list. Unfortunately, most mayonnaise on the market today is made from soybean oil, not the best choice but a necessary compromise in many cases. If you can afford it, you might find a far more expensive mayonnaise made from all olive oil in the gourmet section. Once again, read the label carefully, so that you do not waste extra money on a product where they add a few drops of olive oil to ordinary mayonnaise.

There is another mayonnaise choice. Gourmet cookbooks contain recipes for homemade mayonnaise using olive oil. However, I advise against this unless you can find salmonella-free eggs. Egg farms today are mass-production centers that are breeding grounds for salmonella bacteria in the laying hens. The eggs they produce are safe to eat only if completely cooked. Factory-made mayonnaise is safe because it is sterilized in the bottling process but homemade mayonnaise is not. There is a new process that will destroy salmonella in raw eggs, allowing their safe use. Those treated eggs can now be found only at one supermarket chain and one wholesale restaurant supplier, but check our website www.HippocraticDiet.com for newer information. Until then, compromise on the mass-produced store-bought mayonnaise.

Since you still are in the condiments section, you may want to pick up some pickles or some pickle relish. If you do, read the labels closely and avoid the ones sweetened with sugar.

If you are interested in mustard, most prepared mustards are okay except for the sweetened varieties with added sugar. If you crave the taste of sweetened mustard, add some calorie-free sweetener to prepared mustard.

Are you a ketchup user? Tomatoes do have natural carbohydrates, but most brands of ketchup also contain large amounts of added sugar or high fructose corn syrup. Low-carb ketchup is now available, if you wish.

Avoid the barbecue and steak sauces. Instead, use the calorie-free barbecue sauce recipe found in the recipe section of this book. It is made from smoked chipotle pepper sauce and works well for both steaks and barbecue.

Skip the Worcestershire sauce family entirely. The classic form of Worcestershire sauce contains fermented anchovies. This is one of the few historic forms of free glutamate, or MSG. The newer, cheaper Worcestershire sauces usually contain the chemical form of MSG. Either way, you lose.

You may find the baking and sweetening section nearby. Look for the artificial sweeteners we mentioned earlier. If you do not like artificial sweeteners, consider Stevia, a calorie-free sweetener from an herb. Pick up some unsweetened 100 percent pure baking cocoa. Do not forget to stock up on liquid non-calorie sweetener. Many powdered sweeteners actually add sugar or starch as a "flowing agent." You may also wish to buy a non-calorie brown sugar substitute, but you must be careful when purchasing non-calorie sweeteners. There is at least one well-known brand that uses its brand name on both non-calorie and reduced-calorie sweeteners, so you must read every label and not just rely on a familiar brand name.

You may prefer to get your vegetables in the frozen food or canned food departments. Both are fine, if you are buying pure vegetables. However, be cautious and avoid vegetables with added ingredients. Look out for sugar that is added to certain canned vegetables. In the frozen vegetable department, stay away from vegetables that come with added sauces and, of course, mixtures containing beans, peas or pasta.

Next, you may be ready to visit the meat department of your market. If you live in a big city, you might be lucky enough to find some local independent butcher shops nearby. If you live near a rural area, a local farmer, rancher or packing plant may sell locally raised meat products without injected additives. Otherwise, you are stuck with the large big-box supermarket with its so-called meat department. I say "so-called" because there is a trend for supermarkets to use prepackaged meats. Peek behind the freezer case wall. See if there are people in white coats cutting large sections of meat into small slices or if they are simply opening large cartons of pre-processed food. Try to avoid the chain markets that have their meat cut and packaged in the large processing plants.

Whatever you do, do not buy your meat in those pre-cut restaurant and individual serving packages, whether it is from a supermarket, a home delivery service, or by a mail order. Such portion-controlled meat is highly likely to be infused with a broth that is a devil's brew of free glutamates, preservatives, and other chemicals. They even go so far as to douse their meats with deadly carbon monoxide gas, which prevents the blood in the meat from turning brown and allows old meat to retain a fresh red appearance.

Do not be fooled by advertising that a particular meat product is hormone-free or antibiotic-free. Those are nice attributes providing information about how the animals were raised, but they tell you nothing about what chemicals were added by the meat processor. I have seen packing plants selling *"Amish-raised"* meats where MSG-containing spice mixtures were added to ground sausage. Even products passing the rigorous religious inspection process for a Kosher meat certification may have MSG-containing hydrolyzed vegetable protein added.

Poultry can be just as bad as other products. Fresh poultry markets were once common but are a rarity today. Most poultry sold in supermarkets has been processed hundreds or thousands of miles from where it is being sold. It is then infused with another magic broth. There is one national brand which costs a lot more that is free of this broth. It is worth the extra price and it is a tastier product than the modified chicken, but be careful. The food-processing companies know a good thing when they see it. They now sell alternative, supposedly premium brands of poultry right next to this expensive brand. Their supposedly premium chicken may have all sorts of puffery and claims on the front label but turn it over and you will see that it contains the same magic broth as the cheaper chicken. When you are paying a premium price, you deserve the real product for which you pay extra.

Seafood is another matter. Its hard say which seafood alternative is better. Today, some fish is frozen and sealed at large South American ocean-side fish farms, inland Asian fish farms, or massive foreign refrigerator ships. Other fish is cut and sold at your local supermarket fish counter but usually is no fresher. Most often, those products are simply frozen whole, then thawed at your supermarket before they are put on ice and sold as if fresh. The old-fashioned fish market where fresh products were sold is a rarity, except for a few costal areas where fishing fleets operate.

Remember that the darker the fish, the higher the percentage of healthy fish oil. Shellfish such as crab and lobster is okay, but contains little or no fat. That is why it is so traditional to dip lobster meat in drawn butter. Stay away from the imitation crab and lobster meat. This is usually a cheap whitefish such as pollack or cod, which has been infused with artificial flavoring and MSG.

Canned fish may be okay, depending on what it is. You can get sardines packed in oil without additives. You may want canned kippered herring, which is high in healthy fish oil. Canned salmon works well in some recipes. Avoid fermented anchovies because of the possibility of free glutamate.

Canned tuna is a special case. Healthy tuna packed in olive oil is still available in supermarkets but it is hard to find. Years ago, at the beginning of the low-fat craze, the food companies convinced many people to switch to lighter tuna packed in water. Consumers did so in the mistaken belief that it was a healthier choice. The packers were actually substituting a cheaper variety of fish for the better quality darker tuna. To give it flavor they pack it in hydrolyzed vegetable broth. The real stuff, when you can find it, is sold as a gourmet premium product at about three times the cost of the cheapest canned tuna, but It is worth paying extra for. Read the ingredients list carefully. It should list only tuna and olive oil. If you normally use canned tuna only as an ingredient in tuna salad, you will be pleasantly surprised. MSG-free tuna in olive oil is delicious right out of the can. Adding a bit of this canned tuna to a green salad makes a tasty and well-balanced meal.

Since meat products may still be on your mind, let us talk about the delicatessen section. The deli section can be found in two places. There are the inexpensive prepackaged processed sliced meat products in a refrigerator case, then there is the deli counter where they will slice better quality products to your order.

Surprisingly, I must tell you to avoid the deli counter, unless you have a good relationship with the workers there. The prepackaged products in the refrigerator case all have labels that you can read. The bulk products at the deli counter have labels on the bulk packages, but asking to see each of the labels at a busy deli counter can be a real problem. I have tried, without success, to get this information directly from the food producers. Even though it is not a secret and is readily available to the people behind the counter, these companies would still rather not have you read their labels. This is sad, since many of these producers portray an image of purity and wholesomeness. You would think they would not try to keep this information from your eyes.

If you do buy deli products from the refrigerator case, at least you can take your time and read the fine print of the ingredient label. Very few of these products are free of MSG or hydrolyzed vegetable protein or some other form of free-glutamate. The few that are MSG-free often boast of it on the front label, but you still want to double-check the ingredient list. Some producers are not above saying **MSG-free** on the front of the package while the ingredient list clearly shows hydrolyzed vegetable protein. Others resort to extreme trickery, such as the company that boasts "**No added MSG * * **" on its front label. The words **NO** and **MSG** are highlighted while the word **added** is in small print. You have to search the entire package until you find the * * explained in a footnote at the bottom of the package back in <u>very fine print</u>. It reads "* * *except that found naturally in hydrolyzed vegetable protein*." Of course, the ingredient list does list the hydrolyzed vegetable protein. *What is the average consumer to think?*

If you look hard enough, you will find a few products that

are truly MSG-free, but it takes some work. Many of the cured products, such as ham and bacon, also contain sugar. Try to find the ones with the least amount of sugar, using the Nutrition Facts box.

Cured meat products may also contain preservatives, such as nitrate. These preservatives serve an important function by protecting food from dangerous bacterial spoilage. Unfortunately, some believe they can cause other health problems. This is another one of those areas where you must weigh one health issue against another. It is too lengthy a topic to cover here and does not relate to the obesity issue. However, for those of you who wish to avoid nitrates, be warned. Many food products boast that they do not contain nitrates but, in fact, they use substitute additives that turn into nitrate after being added to food. *It seems as if truth-in-labeling has a long way to go!*

Leaving the deli department, do not forget to shop for dairy products. Traditionally, it had always been the butterfat-containing cream that was recognized as the most significant milk product. An old name for a milk-processing facility was creamery. It was the important cream portion that was vital for the nutritionally rich butter and cheese products. When completely separated, the left-over skim milk portion had other historic uses. These have included being the base for house paint and used as hog feed or slop.

Sorry, but while avoiding sugar, you should avoid milk. Instead, the first thing on your list should be heavy whipping cream. If your market carries it, the best type of whipping cream is pure and fresh. Unfortunately, this can be difficult to find.

Recently, creameries switched to producing ultra-pasteurized cream. The reason for this was pure economics. Ultra-pasteurization is a process that heats the product to a slightly higher temperature than regular pasteurization. This allows the finished product to have a longer shelf life while refrigerated and some products do not need any refrigeration. These ultra-pasteurized products last for months before spoiling. The disadvantage of this method is that the flavor of the product is altered. To compensate, the producers may add various flavor enhancers. Some producers go one step further, also adding thickeners and coloring agents and including less cream in the product. When buying cream, follow the shorter-list rule. If you can find it, buy fresh cream that has been pasteurized but not ultra-pasteurized. If you cannot find this pure product, buy the cream with the shortest ingredient list.

If you wish, buy butter. Avoid butter substitutes. Salted butter is the purest product. Unsalted sweet butter may contain extra additives.

Cheese should be the next item on your list. Whether it comes in a block, sliced, cubed, shredded or grated, real cheese is made with cream, enzymes, and perhaps salt. Sometimes annatto is added for a bright orange color. Some of the grated and shredded cheeses have small amounts of other ingredients added as flowing agents. These flowing agents sometimes contain small amounts of carbohydrate.

Some recipes call for crumpled bleu cheese or feta cheese. If you prefer, you can purchase this product whole and crumple it yourself. By doing this, you will avoid the carbohydrate-containing flowing agent added to the pre-crumpled cheese. The same goes for shredded cheese that ordinarily comes in a shaker box.

Avoid items called *imitation cheese* or *cheese-products*.

They are usually made by substituting vegetable oils for the more costly real cream and may be loaded with other products. Read the Nutrition Facts box and ingredient list on any cheese that you buy.

Cheese is a healthy and nutritious food that has been in use for millennia. It took a beating from the low-fat craze but it is making a comeback. It will be useful in a number of recipes. Cheese cubes are also a handy snack food. One small caution about eating cheese. Some people will find that they become constipated when they eat too much cheese. If this happens to you, modify your cheese use.

Real sour cream is another important product. When you compare the ingredient list on real sour cream to the various imitation forms of light or non-fat sour cream, you will see the difference. The Nutrition Facts boxes will show quite a remarkable contrast, too. There are a number of important recipes that you will find in this book calling for real sour cream. Stock up on it early, since it is allowed during the initiation phase.

Eggs are usually found nearby. Stock up on them. It is amazing that eggs went from being a health food, with the U.S. government recommending that you eat one egg every day to a taboo food with the government recommending that you avoid eggs. They are now back to being a health food and you will even find premium eggs with the chickens fed in a way that increases their eggs' content of healthy omega-3 fatty acid.

As you leave the dairy department, you may want to visit the beverage department and snack department on your way to the check-out cashier. In the beverage department, coffee, tea, and herbal tea are fine. Avoid the pre-mixed flavored instant coffee and tea that often contains sugar. Avoid any powdered beverage next unless it clearly is labeled as zero calories.

If you are a soda drinker, this diet allows reasonable amounts of non-calorie diet soda. Although there are other health concerns with these products, I am not restricting their use for the purposes of this diet. There is even one recipe for "real cream soda" in this book, mixing a small amount of real cream and diet soda. It is a useful thing to try during the initiation phase and many non-soda drinkers love it, since it tastes like an old-fashioned ice cream float.

Non-calorie flavored seltzer and sparkling water are allowed. It is even okay to use those Italian-style flavoring syrups they use in the coffee shops if you can find the sugar-free variety. Despite saying it is permitted to use this wide range of non-calorie beverages, the best beverage is always water. Drink water liberally. If the tap water in your area has an off-taste, consider purchasing bottled water or using a water-filtering pitcher.

Snacks might seem incompatible with dieting, but they are important. Finding satisfying snacks that stay within the limits of this diet gives you the ability to handle special situations. Treat snacks like any other food item. Keep track of them because quantity counts!

One of the best group of foods that are found in the snack section are nuts. These include the true tree nuts, seeds such as sunflower and pumpkin, and peanuts which are actually related to peas and beans. All of them contain a mixture of fat, protein, and carbohydrates. In modest quantities, they are all acceptable on this diet but if you overdo it, you may exceed your carbohydrate allowance.

Many dieters love roasted cashews and almonds but many

have issues with portion control when eating these delicious but healthy snacks. One of the best ways around this is to buy nuts in small bags instead of large cans. Another way that works well is to use small plastic snack bags and measure out the proper amount in advance.

Portion control is easier if you can buy nuts still in the shell. Pistachios, peanuts, and sunflower seeds are readily available in the shell. Taking the time to open each shell individually completely changes your eating pattern with this tasty snack. Remember to read the ingredient list. The only ingredients should be nuts and perhaps salt. Avoid nuts that are coated with anything else. Some nuts come coated with sugar. Many dry-roasted nuts come coated with MSG and other items.

While we are talking about nuts, I should mention nut butters. Real nut butters are nutritionally equal to real nuts. Unfortunately, food processors learned long ago that if they took the peanut oil out of peanuts, they could sell it separately at a high price. They then could grind the peanut residue and mix it with cheap cottonseed or soybean oil, add sugar, and market this imitation product to your children. This has been going on for so long you may have never tasted real peanut butter. Fortunately, there is a movement back to the real thing, with at least one national brand selling real peanut butter. Even better, a few large markets and gourmet shops use a machine that grinds fresh roasted peanuts into pure peanut butter while you watch. There are also some health food shops selling nut butter from more expensive nuts, such as almonds and cashews. Check them out and sample these interesting products.

The last item to consider in the snack department is very different. Unflavored bacon rinds are a common snack food in some places while others turn up their nose at this product. If you eat pork products, try them. They can be crushed and used as a bread crumb substitute in cooking. They can satisfy a craving for a crunchy snack and can be used as a substitute for chips for use with dips. Get them fresh. Stale bacon rinds become rancid and taste bad. Always buy the unflavored variety, which has no MSG.

Now you are ready to head to the cashier. Buying real products instead of imitation products is costly. At first, it may seem that your grocery bills are higher due to buying these more expensive products. With time, you should notice these costs go down because you lose your craving for junk food and you will be buying foods in smaller quantity. Most people find that one balances out the other. Even when it does not, after a few weeks on this diet people do not ever want to go back to the imitation foods. They feel better eating real foods that taste so much better.

During your first few visits to the grocery store, prepare for the extra time that it will take to shop. This is because you are reading label after label until you find satisfactory products. Once you become familiar with what works and what does not work, this will become easier and your shopping time will return to normal.

The one thing that will change forever will be your appreciation of real food.

12

Eating Out and Traveling

When you are just starting your plan, the thought about eating away from home can be scary. At home you have control over your environment, but questions arise when you will have to eat away from home. Some problems are easily solved while others pose a real dilemma. This chapter deals with strategies that many different people have developed. Questions about eating out and traveling are probably the most frequent issue that comes up as new dieters join our support groups. Fortunately, the wisdom within the group often prevails. There is generally another group member who has faced something similar and will explain how she or he did it. This chapter is a compilation of various strategies that have come from these groups. Your situation may not be exactly the same, but you may be able to glean enough from their wisdom to find the answer to your problem.

Avoid Eating Out

This is the simplest strategy of them all. It may seem rather limited, unless you ask yourself, "Do I really need to eat out on this occasion?" Many times, we choose to eat out because it seems like the simplest alternative. If you really do not need to, do not do it and you avoid any conflict.

Get to Pick the Spot

When going out with a group, it pays to be assertive. Sometimes, groups have a hard time deciding where to go and just by being assertive, you can provide an answer. At other times, you may need to be more forceful and state that you can only go if certain places are avoided. Finally, if with friends, play the diet card. Explain that you are on a restricted diet and only particular places will meet your needs.

Skip It

One dieter works in an environment where the staff orders out for pizza the same day each week. Her strategy is to fast that day every week. Because she now fasts easily, she does not feel deprived by missing a meal and not joining her colleagues.

Avoid Buffets

You may be able to pick the right foods from a buffet but it is difficult. All-you-can-eat restaurants make their money by emphasizing cheap food. That means that much of what they put out is high in carbohydrate. If they serve meat or chicken, it is likely to be a cheaper cut made tastier with MSG. An additional trap is that you may feel compelled to get your money's worth when eating at this type of restaurant. These are dangerous places for dieters and best avoided.

Ask for a Take-Home Box

Instead of waiting until the end of the meal, have a take-home container brought to you when your food comes to the table. Put the excess food into the box and just leave the part you should eat on your plate.

Split a Meal

If you are eating out with another light eater or dieter, splitting a meal is a sensible strategy. Most restaurants will go along with it.

Hold the Sides

Be sure to clearly tell your waiter or waitress that you do not want the potatoes, muffins, bread, or other items that they include as side orders with your dinner. Surprisingly, some may argue with you, so be assertive. Perhaps they think they are doing you a favor by bringing all the food you paid for.

Ask for Alternative Side Dishes

The smarter waiters and waitresses will want to cooperate with you and provide alternatives, even when they may not be listed on the menu. Let them know you would be happy to pay a small extra charge to replace the potatoes with a vegetable.

Order Eggs

Some restaurants have a 24-hour breakfast policy. See if

you can order eggs, no matter what time of day it is. Try to order them without extra items you do not want to eat.

Ask for a Side Order

Chain restaurants may be slaves to their computer systems. They may resist accepting an order for eggs without the associated pancakes and other trappings, if it is ordered as a main course. However, the waiter often has an alternative of putting in an order as a side order for just the specific item you want. Ask for it.

Ask for Alternative Menus

Many restaurant chains have alternative menus for those with particular dietary needs. These may be menus for diabetics, children's menus, senior menus, menus for people with gluten restrictions, and menus for dieters. Do not be afraid to ask about them, all they can say is no. If you are neither a senior nor a child, some waitresses will think you are being cheap by ordering from a special menu. Explain that you are diabetic. Show a diabetic bracelet, if necessary.

You may wish to have your doctor sign a small card like the one shown below. Carry it with you for argumentative waiters. I provide this for dieters under my care and it seems to work.

Mary Smith
_____ is on a restricted diet for medical reasons and may be unable to consume your standard meal portions. When dining at your restaurant, your cooperation will be appreciated. Please assist by allowing her/him to order senior, children's, half or side portions when available.
Thank you for your help.

Jane Doe, M.D.

When used, dieters have received complete cooperation.

Order Appetizers

An appetizer portion may be perfect for your main course. If you are with a group, you may even get them to order multiple appetizer platters for themselves, instead of a main course. Some Spanish-style restaurants specialize in serving a variety of *tapas,* tasty Mediterranean appetizer dishes.

Throw Away the Bun

At a fast-food chain, you may be forced to order a small salad and small burger. Take it and toss out the bun. Many people have done it before you. At a conference where they serve box lunches, carrying a plastic fork can be handy for eating the contents of the sandwiches.

Order Salads

Many restaurants feature Chef's salad and Cobb's salad. These are often reasonable choices except for the portion sizes. Split them or put half into a take-out container.

Ask for a Half-Size

Some restaurants have half-size salads available but do not list them prominently. Ask if they do.

Hold the Croutons

Let your waiter know what you do not want on your salad in advance rather than have to pick things out once the salad has been brought to you.

Ask for Olive Oil

Do not take a chance on their pre-mixed salad dressing. Ask for oil and vinegar, but make it clear you do not want the house pre-mixed version. Some restaurants normally have this option available, but all restaurants have some sort of oil in the kitchen that they can bring to you.

Order Bleu Cheese Dressing

If you must use their dressing, bleu cheese is often the best choice.

Carry your own Salad Dressing

This is more difficult for a man but many women have told me that they take a small container with their homemade salad dressing in their handbag. They asked for their salad without dressing and explain that they have a need for their own dressing. According to them, no one has ever objected.

Carry Nuts and Cheese

This is a great travel strategy that may enable you to skip stopping at airport and roadside restaurants. Bags of nuts are also handy in a hotel room or at a conference where you can not eat their lunch.

Leave the Shells on Hard-boiled Eggs.

Hard-boiled eggs that have been chilled in your refrigerator and with the shell still intact usually keep well when traveling.

Stay with Friends or Relatives

If you have a choice of staying in a home-like environment where you can have refrigerator privileges, this may be easier then staying at a hotel. Be sure that your host understands and will be supportive.

<u>*Do Not*</u> *Stay with Friends or Relatives*

Sometimes, it is easier to do just the opposite. If you plan a trip to visit family but are afraid that they will not be cooperative, staying elsewhere may be the best strategy for you. When making this decision, you know your family better than anyone else .

Stay at a Hotel with a Refrigerator

An in-room refrigerator is handy and allows you to pick up a few items, such as real cream and cheese cubes and store them in your room.

Stay at a Hotel with a Hot Breakfast

Chapter 12   Eating Out and Traveling

Many hotels include a breakfast with the price of a room, but it is often a high-carbohydrate Continental breakfast with few choices. However, some hotels include a hot breakfast, usually featuring items such as eggs and breakfast meats. Even if you ordinarily skip breakfast at home, this may help you get through your day's events without being frustrated when a sensible lunch is difficult to obtain.

Walk

Your diet and your activity level are often disrupted by travel. If you are some place that allows you to safely walk about, consider doing some extra walking while staying at your hotel.

Compromise on Half and Half.

If you drink coffee when you are out, the "cream" they bring you is either half-and-half or that dreaded high-carbohydrate concoction called *creamer*. Although half-and-half is not recommended for home use, it is a reasonable compromise when away from home. You may want to carry some of those little tubs of half-and-half with you. They require no refrigeration and are useful in hotels which supply sugary powdered creamer for those in-room coffee makers.

Check Out Restaurants Online

Knowing what is nearby and what their menus are before you arrive in a strange city can take away some of your concerns. If you are at a conference and going out with a group for dinner, knowing the choices gives you the upper-hand in picking a sensible restaurant.

Offer to Cook for Your Host

When staying with family see if you can arrange to be the cook during the visit. This allows you to be sure that appropriate dishes will be available to you.

Plan Ahead

The anticipation of coping with travel produces unneeded anxiety. Whatever strategy you select, the act of planning ahead is helpful in relieving that stress. Plan to bring your testing supplies and logs <u>and use them</u>.

Enjoy Yourself

Some people are nervous when they return from a trip. They are certain that they did something so horrible that they have gained weight. They are usually wrong and have either held steady or continued to lose weight during their travels. There may be times that you will be tempted to do things you would not do at home. Allow yourself the freedom to be human, but keep testing to see when you have made a mistake. **Just do not do anything really stupid.** *And if you do, just go back to the initiation phase of the plan, monitor yourself closely and get back on track.*

If you are on vacation, try to enjoy yourself without obsessing beforehand.

You will handle it better than you anticipate!

13

Accepting the Slimmer You

Losing weight means different things to different people. Since most type 2 diabetics need to lose weight, they share these experiences with all dieters. Your weight is the outward marker of regaining health. Your friends and coworkers might have been unaware of your diabetes, but a change in weight is seen by others. One person might lose thirty pounds and be pleased with it. Another person may lose one hundred and thirty pounds and have his life totally changed. Being overweight is more than just a question of diet and exercise. There are also tie-ins to significant emotional issues. Whole books have been written about the emotional burden of being overweight; yet, diet books often gloss over this issue.

Renewing Hope

No overweight person ever wanted to be that way. The people who have come to see me have all tried many other methods and at many different times in their life. They are the survivors. Something made them decide to try one last time, one more time, and try something different. Often it was seeing a friend or acquaintance successfully lose weight they had been unable to do before. That gave them the one tool that every dieter needs, *hope*. **Hope** *is a necessary tool when dieting.*

Accepting Success

Unfortunately, many dieters have held that hope before, only to have it dashed by an ineffective diet. Surgery, pills, exercise plans all claim to hold the answer to a cure. When these do not work, the victim is blamed. In most cases, it is the victim blaming herself. She develops an attitude that she is born to be fat. At that point, she may give up on herself. She may accept a stereotype. You know them. *The jolly fat lady. The fat but tough lady. The sexy fat lady.* Men, too, accept similar stereotypes. *Stout. Good old boy.*

Accepting these stereotypes is one defense against what we may feel is a self-failure. If we accept a false belief that we are incapable of losing weight, then we do not have to try anymore, only to fail once again. Dashed hopes from repeated failure are painful. Even a person who only needs to lose twenty pounds may feel this. A person who needs to lose sixty or eighty pounds often feels inadequate. One person may put this inadequacy in a compartment. She may feel inadequate about her physique but emphasize her other qualities. Another person may have this feeling of failure extend to other parts of his life. Unfortunately, the world can be unkind. Jokes, ridicule, job discrimination, and other negative events make overweight persons feel that they are less worthy than others.

As you successfully lose weight on this diet, you should be pleased. However, some people will be pleased and confused at the same time. If you have struggled with failure for many years, you may be confused by success. It is not you. It is not who you are supposed to be. It will not work. You are waiting for the other shoe to drop.

Learning to accept the slim you hidden under that extra fat is easier said than done. You need to get your mind around your victory. *Accept good things that are happening to you.*

Celebrate Your Success

Chart your weight-loss as well as your improvement in glucose control. Celebrate every victory. Everyone has little milestones, things they could not do before that they find they can do with weight loss. These will be different for every individual but meaningful for everyone. What these milestones are depends on who you are and how much you have to lose. Some examples have been the following:

- Having your physician call you with normal test results
- Painting your toenails you had not been able to reach
- Wearing your teenage daughter's jeans
- Sitting comfortably in an airline seat
- Crossing your legs comfortably
- Going up and down stairs without being short of breath
- Buying clothes in the regular department

This list could go on, but you get the idea. There will be some point where you find yourself doing something you were not able to do before dieting. This will occur long before you reach any final goal. The experience will be very satisfying because it shows you are on the road that you always hoped you could be on. *Milestones reinforce your belief in success.*

Chapter 13   *Accepting the Slimmer You*

Be Sensible about Activity

Reasonable exercise is part of any weight-loss program. It is over-estimated in its ability to take off pounds but under-estimated in its ability to improve your health and self-esteem. You may have to start out very slowly. Water exercises, yoga, and Tai-Chi are some methods which can increase your range of motion without being too strenuous. Gradually, you can increase your activity. Hippocrates had a simple suggestion *"Do things with those younger than yourself."* That is always a good method for increasing your activity level. **Activity can make you feel better about yourself.**

Dreams may be Doable

I always use the word *dream* in questioning people about their goals. People often come in hoping to lose twenty pounds, because they do not think they are capable of losing what they really want to lose. That is why I ask what their dream weight is. That might be what they weighed on their wedding day or at their high school graduation. They have given up hope of reaching it again. For many people, that dream weight may still be a realistic goal, but they had given up on themselves. Now, once they see that they can successfully lose weight they regain the ability to dream. **Allow yourself to realize that dreams can be realistic.**

Look Your Best

For some people, this is frightening. Some people are afraid that looking good will bring unwanted advances from others. Others may be reminded of attractive but shallow people who they know. Some may be scared that their good looks will frighten an insecure spouse. Some people just do not want to be noticed. *Look good, you deserve it.*

You Can Win at Many Things

If your self-image about your weight extended to other parts of your life, changing your weight can open doors for you. These doors were not locked by others, but by you, yourself. Losing weight, getting a new wardrobe and a new hairstyle to go with the new look can be just the right steps for some. Going back to school, applying for a better job, reaching out for new relationships are all possible next steps. *Expand your horizons.*

Don't be Alone

Are you doing this all on your own? If you can find support, you will do better. This is not a new idea. Call them support groups or diet clubs, they go back over a century. During the time it takes you to diet, many things can happen. You can have good and bad days. Some of these will be related to diet, others will be completely unrelated events but ones that can lead you to destructive emotional eating. Having others involved can and does help. There are also negative people around you, who may do things to sabotage your dieting. Having a support group is one defense against these negative folks. *Accept the support and help of others.*

Successful Dieters Can Help Each Other.

What kind of support group do you need? For most people, any type of diet support group will work as long as it is based on honesty and sincerity. It may be a circle of friends who decide to begin dieting and controlling their diabetes together. It may be a group at your workplace or your place of worship. *It should not be a commercial group selling diet products.*

There are two nonprofit groups that have helped people with weight problems for half a century. These are Overeaters Anonymous and TOPS. These groups have helped many thousands of women and men. They have different approaches to the problem, with Overeaters Anonymous focusing more on the emotional issues of being overweight and TOPS dealing more with the mechanical issue of dieting. If you need further support, both can be a resource. If you go to such a group, seek out the people who have been successful. Ideally, find someone like yourself, a type 2 diabetic who has successfully lost weight without pills or surgery. *Stick with the winners.*

Check their websites to find a group near you

Overeaters Anonymous
WWW.OA.ORG

TOPS
WWW.TOPS.ORG

Find Support Right Around You

There is an old story about a sailing ship that was stuck because of calm winds. Its crew and passengers were running out of drinking water. Seeing a steamship come into view, they signaled for water. The steamship replied *"CAST DOWN YOUR BUCKET WHERE YOU ARE!"*

Although at sea, they had not realized that they were at the mouth of a large river. The outflow meant that the very water they were sailing upon was fresh to drink. Often, you can find support from those around you. I consider these people the *real supporters*. As you lose weight, they provide you with positive feedback and acceptance. Learn to accept their help. Some people may fear disappointing these supporters and will reject their genuine help. *You cannot disappoint your real supporters because they accept you for who you are.* They are there for you during struggles you may be having. **Embrace your real supporters. "Cast down your bucket where you are."**

Good Friends Don't Mean to Harm

You live in a world where there are many people. Do not let others hurt you while you are reshaping yourself, both literally and figuratively. There will be some around you who I call *helpful friends.* They often give you mixed messages. They probably mean no harm but . . .

Ignore Bad Messages but Accept Good Intent.

Chapter 13   *Accepting the Slimmer You*

Some Folks Talk Just to Hear Themselves

There are other folks around you who can be quite harmful. Some are casual observers, who really do not care about you but still can make harmful remarks. They may be ignorant or think that they are funny. Like the last group, they too, are best ignored. *Learn to ignore ignorance.*

Other Folks are Threatened by Your Success

Finally, there are the truly nasty ones. They bring you sugar cookies when they know you are diabetic. They criticize whatever methods of diet you are using, saying it can not be healthy for you. They tell you that you look terrible as you become slimmer. They do all these things wearing a smile and saying that they mean it in your best interest. *These people have problems of their own.* Sometimes they are overweight and resent it when someone else is successful at losing weight. They may feel that your success highlights their own failures. *Pity the Nasty Folks. They have Problems of Their Own.*

Put yourself first.

Think of this as "healthy selfishness." When we are young, we are often taught to not be selfish. We loathe the self-centered person who thinks of no one else. Unfortunately, this can be overdone. It can lead to self-loathing and low self-esteem.

Can you recall the speech the stewardess gives when you are on a plane? She says "If you are flying with a small child and the plane is depressurized, put on your own oxygen mask first." When I ask parents to recall this speech, they often get it backwards. It is instinct to help your child first. That is the very reason the airlines make you listen to this speech every time you fly. Were you to put your child 's mask on first, you would pass out and be unable to be of further help. By putting yourself first, you not only save yourself, but you are also able to save your child.

Hillel was a Jewish rabbi and scholar who lived when Christ was young. He taught about this healthy selfishness in the following words:

- *If I am not for myself, who is for me?*
- *When I am (only) for myself, what am I?*
- *If not now, when?*

Have you ever paid more attention to not offending someone who was pushing food on you, rather than to your own needs as a diabetic? There are times you must be selfish! This does not mean that you are a bad person. It is right to consider others, but not before yourself.

If I am not for myself, who is for me?

Points for Success

- *<u>Hope</u> is a necessary tool when dieting.*
- *Accept good things that are happening to you.*
- *Milestones reinforce your belief in success.*
- *Activity can make you feel better about yourself.*
- *Allow yourself to realize that dreams can be realistic.*
- *Look good, you deserve it.*
- *Expand your horizons.*
- *Accept the support and help of others.*
- *Stick with the winners.*
- *Embrace your real supporters.*
  "Cast down your bucket where you are."
- *Ignore bad messages, but accept good intent.*
- *Learn to ignore ignorance.*
- *Pity the nasty folks. They have problems of their own.*
- *If I am not for myself, who will be?*

14

Maintaining Your Recovery

When my patients see that they are reversing their diabetes and losing weight successfully on this plan, they begin to ask questions about maintaining that recovery. I answer that they will not need me to provide a maintenance plan because when they reach that point, they will have developed their own individual plans for how to live their lives. As you first read this, you may wonder what this means, but after you have been both controlling your diabetes and losing weight for a few weeks you will understand.

This is not simply a plan or a diet; you have been changing your lifestyle. Look back at what you have already done. If you now have normal glucose readings and have been losing weight, you have already taken important steps in making this change:

- Your maintenance plan began the day you cleaned your cupboards of harmful faux foods. That action was a first step in declaring your independence from foods that may harm you.

- The next step that you took was to greatly reduce your carbohydrate intake. You learned that excess carbohydrates are always the enemy of controlling diabetes.

- As you changed the mixture of foods you were eating, you gained a better understanding of the need for balance within your diet.

- You kept close watch on your food intake, your metabolic state, and your weight. Doing this helped you learn what works for you. Your close monitoring of blood sugar paid off.

- You began to feel better physically, and your energy level changed.

- As you began to lose weight, you increased your activity level in a way that was sensible for you.

- Working with your doctor, you saw your test results improve, while your need for medication decreased. You learned that you have the power to prevent or control disease--even when problems have already begun.

- As you learned that you were not helpless or a failure in controlling your diabetes and your weight, your self-esteem and outlook on life improved.

- You learned that rigid mealtimes were not required when your body had enough energy.

- You found that as your body became more efficient, your energy needs were reduced and you needed to make adjustments to your diet to maintain a steady course.

- You may have discovered sensitivities to certain foods which made you feel bad.

- You may have discovered "trigger foods" that set you off on an eating binge.

- You may have made some mistakes, but you learned from them. You developed the habit of not feeling sorry for yourself with each mistake you made. Instead, you learned to recognize what your weaknesses were, both metabolically and emotionally.

- You discovered that brief fasts are one way to reset your metabolism at times when you have gone astray.

- You may have noticed that there is more to controlling diabetes and losing weight then simply shedding fat as your body remodeled itself.

- You became optimistic about your future as you began to look, act, and feel younger.

These are accomplishments for which you can be proud. Congratulate yourself for what you have already done. This is a good time to put aside irrational fears based upon previous experiences when you may have regained weight after losing some. Re-read the list of what you have already done. You have learned to use tools that will see you through this next stage.

Some people call this "maintenance," but I prefer to think of it as leveling off. Consider a pilot who has successfully taken off in an airliner. Next, she navigated successfully to her destination. She made some normal course corrections accurately during the journey and used her gauges to let her know how she was doing. As the plane burned fuel, it became lighter and ran more efficiently. The pilot adjusted for these changes as she went along. When the destination was in sight, she followed a specific path to come back to earth and keep the landing smooth. Because each aircraft has different characteristics and conditions vary, her landing may not have been the same as another's. Once she had landed, she taxied to the terminal gate where she could shut down the engines and relax.

When you are ready to level off, you too will have successfully taken off, followed a path, made adjustments and now have your destination in sight. It is the time for you to successfully land. You have the knowledge and experience to do it, if you look back at what you have done so far.

If you stay up in the air, your journey is not complete. Leveling off is a process that takes certain steps. Like the pilot's steps, these may not be the identical for everyone. Follow these general steps to guide you:

- **Do not dream of going back to your old eating habits or you will keep yourself in a never-ending pattern, flying in circles but never reaching your destination**. Once again, remember the insanity of repeating the same old mistakes and expecting them to come out differently.

Expecting to successfully lose weight, reverse your diabetes but then return to the eating pattern that created your problem fits that definition of insanity.

- **Re-evaluate your goal.** If you had to shed a lot of weight, your body has been going through significant remodeling. You first set your goal as if the amount of muscle and bone would not change. If you had a considerable amount to lose, more change could be taking place. All that extra muscle and bone needed to carry your extra weight is no longer needed and may have reduced. On the other hand, your higher activity level may have created more muscle and stronger bones in other places. If these changes are occurring, consider a re-evaluation to decide on a long-term target weight.

- **Plan a steeper flight path before leveling off.** As you begin to shift your body to a steady state, it will regain some short-term storage. When you started to diet, you rid yourself of glycogen and its associated water. That told your body to burn stored fat. As you level off, it is normal for your body to rebuild some of that glycogen. Allow yourself a few pounds for that purpose. Everyone will differ, but I suggest allowing your weight-loss diet to continue about four to six pounds below your goal. As your body rebuilds its stored short-term glycogen, this natural readjustment should level you off at your goal.

- **Stay in touch with your doctor.** This is particularly important if you were started or stopped on any medication while dieting. Recheck baseline lab tests. Continue to closely monitor your blood sugar and filling in your log.

- **Continue to avoid flavor-enhancers.** Free glutamates such as MSG have been our focus because they are overeating triggers. Continue to avoid them.

- **Continue to avoid high-sugar foods.** Today, the average American consumes about <u>twenty-five times as much sugar</u> as did Americans at the time of the American Revolution. Since you may have acquired a high-sugar taste, continue to use artificial sweeteners as long as you need them. Your body has learned to associate the sugar taste with the brief good feeling from the sugar rush.

  As you continue to develop into a sugar-free person this association will weaken and with time, your body will no longer demand over-sweetened foods. If you are raising children, try not to get them hooked on the need for that sweetness. Instead, they will learn to appreciate sweet foods as the special treat that they should be.

- **Add foods gradually.** By adding foods one at a time, you can discover if you are sensitive to certain foods and learn to avoid those foods. Watch for foods that cause a spike in your blood sugar. You may have been suffering from a food sensitivity, irritable bowel syndrome or celiac disease and not even known it. Some people might feel better as their conditions respond favorably to the simpler, purer foods they are now eating. By adding foods slowly, you will be aware of reactions to particular foods.

- **Watch out for and accept your food addictions.** Some people were overweight simply because they ate too much, but others may have been changed by their overeating. Some people will have become actual food addicts, where the chemistry of certain foods triggered a cascade of both biochemical and psychological events that caused them to eat even more.

  One person may decide to eat one chocolate chip cookie and be perfectly okay while another will find she has eaten the whole plate of cookies before the evening is over. She was not bad or weak-willed. Instead, she had a food addiction that was triggered by that one cookie and she should totally avoid that trigger food in the future. The person who was able to eat the cookie should not be smug about it. Although not a trigger for her, some other food might be. That is another reason to add new foods one at a time. It helps identify problem foods that create these addiction issues for you

- **Be alert to the presence of other contaminants.** There are many other substances found in our food that are currently allowed by lax government watchdogs. Some have other potential for harm but have not been banned because of incomplete scientific data, bureaucratic foot-dragging, and misleading information from the food industry. Although these may not be diet-busters, if they have the potential to harm you and your family, ask yourself if you really want them in your food.

- **Continue your activity level.** Hopefully, you have developed an exercise pattern that you really enjoy, not one you glumly dread because it is the "right thing" to do.

- **Continue to track your food intake, your weight and your blood sugar.** Do this as closely as when you were dieting for the first few months. Compare these to your A1c. You will be able to spot some patterns that are danger spots for you.

- **Fast periodically, even if you do not need to lose weight.** This will help insure that the energy pathways you re-opened during this diet continue to stay open. Recently, cardiology researchers studied members of the Church of Jesus Christ of Latter-Day Saints (Mormons) and discovered that those who fast monthly for religious purposes are healthier.

- **Eat less than the government tells you to.** Most dietary guidelines the U.S. Government issues are too generous. They are set with wide safety margins to prevent malnutrition and are a very real factor in over-feeding many people with more calories than they actually need. After World War II, a remarkable thing happened. The devastation of war created food shortages throughout Europe. These shortages continued for several years until the United States intervened and provided massive aid through the Marshall Plan. While Europe was short on food, death rates fell. This phenomena has been duplicated in the laboratory time and again. Eating a little less lengthens life.

- **Plan your maintenance calories.** Since you are not going to attempt to eat as much as you did before, how much should you eat? Personalize your food intake to your needs. Start by going back and reviewing your daily logs. The records you have been keeping should tell you what your energy need is. Look for the time just before you began leveling off. Perhaps you were eating about 800 kilocalories each day but your rate of weight loss had dropped to a pound each week for several weeks. One pound weight loss each week is roughly equal to an energy deficit of about 600 kilocalories each day. Add that 600 to the 800 you were eating and that brings you to about 1,400 kilocalories per day to maintain a steady weight.

- Whatever your number is, it is more likely to be correct than the government's one-size-fits-all recommendation. As you level off, try it and see if this amount of food will keep your weight steady. Research suggests that keeping your food intake at the level that maintains your weight **and no more** is associated with good health and longevity.

- **Eat locally.** Shop at farmers' markets and grow some of your food, if you can. Even city apartment dwellers can grow small window-box and balcony gardens. Knowing who grows your food goes a long way to assuring its freshness and purity. It is also the right thing to do ecologically, since the food you eat will not have been shipped thousands of miles to get to you.

Learn about getting real food
from local farmers at
www.localharvest.org

- **Eat seasonally.** The ancient advice of Ecclesiastes is still worthwhile today. "A season is set for everything...." Today, with most of us far removed from agriculture, we forget this and demand foods out of season.

  Not so long ago we could look forward to the fall, when we could expect to eat fresh, crisp apples. There is an old religious practice of offering a special prayer of thanksgiving the first time you eat a particular fruit or vegetable each year. This simple and joyous practice expresses gratitude for reaching that season. If you visit an orchard when fruit has ripened, you will understand this. The appreciation for nature's wonders and gratitude for enjoying special foods in season simply is not the same when a New Yorker can buy a fresh apple flown in from New Zealand in the spring. Eating seasonally helps your body regulate itself and makes you appreciate the bounty available to you.

- **Eat traditionally.** Selective breeding is a powerful tool that has been used sparingly by agriculturalists for millennia. Over time, implemented slowly, it has helped the human food supply to expand and improve. Today, we see our food changing at a dizzying rate. Massive research has changed this selection process and has been quickened even further by genetic engineering. Some of these new products may prove useful but others could be dangerous.

Time answers many such questions but today chemical companies and food processors have banded together to create foods that offer the most short-term profit for them. Whether it is turkeys bred to grotesque shapes to vary the balance of their meat, apples that grow to the portion size of a softball, or grain that produces its own internal insecticide, a few years of lab study is often inadequate to show all the potential drawbacks. Look for "heritage foods" whenever you can find them. Many small farmers are going back to these, creating a niche market not served by the giant producers.

- **Learn about your own true heritage.** Our nation is a vast melting pot. Even if your genetic roots can be traced back to a single group, it is unlikely that your food traditions are as pure. Many cultures based their traditional food choices on a combination of availability and health. Genetic traits sometimes play a powerful role in the development of food traditions.

    For example, there are cultures that turn milk into fermented kefir or yogurt. This strategy makes sense in parts of the world where lactose intolerance is common, such as Africa and the Mediterranean region. Otherwise, the dairy product would cause gas and diarrhea for those carrying this gene. However, it would not serve the same purpose in Holland or Germany, where this genetic problem is uncommon.

    When you investigate traditional foods, be careful which tradition you use. Foods that became "traditional" during a period of deprivation or limitation are not a good choice. One example is *Indian Fry Bread.* Today, this supposedly traditional food is found at many Native American gatherings. It is not truly traditional, but instead came into use when tribes were forced from their ancestral homes and provided rations of flour and lard by the government. Look back far enough as you search your heritage for foods from good times.

- **Make exceptions for _very special occasions_.** It may be that you are attending your daughter's wedding or your grandparents' fiftieth anniversary. These are not everyday events, and you may feel that you should have a slice of a cake you would otherwise avoid. Okay, you are human and if you decide to do something like that, have a plan. **Do not guilt yourself into saying "I broke my own rules so I may as well go all the way."**

  Instead, be ready to adjust to compensate for going off track and enjoy the special event. Monitor your sugar closely and do not let it get out of control. As you recover from diabetes, you may find that you have regained the ability to tolerate occasional small deviations, but be careful. Learn to consider these decisions and have a plan to quickly resume your healthy behavior. **If you choose to do this, do not do it too often. It is easy to become complacent after doing this once without a problem**. If you do this often, you could revert to a pattern of poor glucose control requiring a return to medication. You may also experience yo-yo dieting, constantly regaining and re-dieting in an unhealthy pattern.

- **Think about your looks wisely.** If you have been increasing activity and exercise, you may be pleasantly surprised as you tightened up. For some, stretched skin may appear less attractive and a reminder of your overweight old self. Enjoy your healthier, new-found body, even if you worry that it is not perfect. Those around you may be telling you how good you look. Accept their compliments, and do not rush to extreme measures.

  Do not try medications or make-up that promises to rid you of wrinkles. This may harm you by irritating your skin to puff it out, not a healthy state. If you are considering having a cosmetic surgeon tighten your skin to match your leaner body, wait a bit. I am not against such cosmetic surgery, so long as you make such a decision slowly and wisely. First, continue to exercise and maintain your new weight for a year or more. Be sure that the person offering to provide such cosmetic surgery is fully residency-trained and Board-Certified in Plastic Surgery. Be sure that you have a long talk with the surgeon before you decide to proceed. The best surgeons will want to be sure that you are realistic and will benefit before they agree to proceed.

- **Help others who need to reverse diabetes or to lose weight.** This action is not purely altruistic. By using your personal experience to help others, you will be reinforcing your own healthy behavior. There are many ways to do this. You may be an example for your family. You may be a support system for friends who are trying to lose weight. You could form a weight-loss support group with acquaintances at your workplace or place of worship. You may ask your doctor about forming a support group within the diabetes clinic. You might attend a nonprofit weight-loss support group, such as TOPS or Overeaters Anonymous. Whichever way you do it, you can feel good about helping another person while actually also helping yourself.

All of these recommendations are not a "maintenance diet" but lifestyle changes. Because of individual differences, there can not be one fixed diet for everyone. I recommend that you use a process of finding the food mix that works best for you.

Start by reviewing the weight-loss diet you just completed. You should have been getting an adequate foundation of protein and fat. You may increase your protein moderately. As you begin to increase your carbohydrate intake, do so mostly in the form of vegetables, peas, and beans. Try modest amounts of fruit that is in season. If you find yourself increasing your fat intake, do so with healthy ones, such as olive oil. Try small amounts of milk or yogurt. Keep things made from grains among the last additions to your diet.

- **Use your experience with your food diary to estimate the energy you need as you vary your diet.** Remember to add foods one at a time. Give each new food a few days and watch your reaction. Foods that cause you to eat more than intended may be trigger foods and you should avoid them.

- **Foods that cause gastrointestinal distress should be noted and avoided.** If you discover some, you may have a food allergy, a food sensitivity or a disorder such as *Irritable Bowel Syndrome* or *Celiac Disease*.

If you suspect such a problem, check with your doctor or a gastroenterologist. Special support groups can provide you more information help you to learn what foods to avoid. You may not have noticed the connection before. Now, you feel better on a limited diet while losing weight. As you add certain foods back, the difference may be noticeable.

For many, this process may result in what I call a
Modified Mediterranean-Style Diet

Much has been written about the health benefits of the so-called *Mediterranean Diet* in recent years, but what does it really mean? Since the diet of nations bordering the Mediterranean Sea varies widely, some nutritionists attempt to rationalize the discredited USDA food pyramid by using similar food combinations to describe Mediterranean eating habits. In fact, some of the diets they describe as supposedly representative are from poor regions that rely heavily on cheap grains. Although olive oil is synonymous with a healthy Mediterranean diet, the average consumption of olive oil can vary by a factor of ten or twenty times between different parts of the Mediterranean. To avoid confusion with these other diets, I use the term *"Modified Mediterranean-Style Diet,"* relying on certain features of food consumption in the Greek Isles.

The wonderful diet of that region is a result of Greek geography. The rugged terrain of the Greek Isles makes the olive tree a preferred agricultural crop and a major

continued

food source. The olive became a source of great wealth in ancient times as the Greeks exported large quantities of this healthy oil throughout the ancient world.

Today, the average consumption of olive oil per person in Greece is more than twenty times that of the average American. Looking at olive oil alone, an average Greek may consume almost a third of their energy intake from this healthy oil. In addition, the Mediterranean Sea surrounding the Greek Isles provides the wealth of fresh fish that is another important part of the Greek eating tradition.

In addition to the fat coming from olive oil, Greeks consume other fats from fish, nuts, meat, cheese and other dairy products. This total of all these fats is well above the 30 percent energy recommendation from fat that heart experts talk about in the United States. Yet Greeks have a lower level of heart disease than we do here in America. The reason is the positive benefit of a diet high in olive oil, fish, and nuts as is found in Greece.

Protein from fish, meat and eggs is present in moderate amounts, but what about carbohydrate? Simply put, a diet with this higher percentage of healthy fat has to displace something. In this case, healthy fat replaces carbohydrates for energy intake in a way that reduces the total amount of carbohydrates eaten.

Next, what types of carbohydrates do I recommend? Mixtures of vegetables including peas and beans with limited amounts of whole grain are the healthiest carbohydrate mixture. However, if you who were previously addicted to carbohydrates, be cautious, some of these may be trigger foods for you.

Finally, allow yourself modest amounts of high sugar foods, primarily from fresh fruit in season. The very last items to cautiously sample are sweetened foods, in very small amounts. Items such as pastries covered with honey should be reserved for holidays and other festive occasions.

By monitoring your blood glucose carefully, you can tell what, how much and how often you can tolerate these additions to your diet.

There is another important issue in maintaining you recovery. *If maintaining ketosis gave you a feeling of well-being and mental clarity, keep close watch on yourself and your mental state.* If you begin to notice a return to your old self, you may be sensing brain chemistry changes as you leave ketosis. If this occurs, you should determine how you can maintain your healthier state **without further weight-loss**. You do not want to join the ranks of those suffering from anorexia, people who starve themselves by continually dieting. If you need to deal with this issue, I can suggest three strategies, but ask you to examine each of these with your physician and only use them with his or her supervision:

1. **Try to maintain this mental balance through periodic brief fasts.** If you attempt this, watch your weight to be sure you do not overdo it.

2. **Follow a ketogenic diet that is <u>not</u> intended to reduce weight.** These higher-fat diets are sometimes called Inuit or Eskimo diets, because native people of the far north traditionally ate like this. They did not have health problems until "civilization" radically changed their diets. Another group who continues to follow a high-fat diet are certain nomadic shepherds of central Asia, noted for living longer than most people elsewhere.

   Such diets require you to keep your carbohydrate level as low as it was when you were losing weight but increase the energy in your diet by increasing the healthiest fats, such as olive oil, fish, foods with higher levels of omega-3 fatty acids, and omega-3 supplements. Have your physician check your lipid levels to verify that you are doing this in a way that will not cause negative changes in your cholesterol.

3. **Consider anti-depressant medication.** The changes in your brain chemistry from your weight-loss and ketosis may have helped you overcome a case of clinical depression. If getting off ketogenic diet triggers a return to depression and is not amenable to other strategies, work with your physician to find a medication that is right for you. Be careful, for some anti-depressant medications trigger both an increase in glucose levels and cause significant weight-gain.

These last three strategies are not general suggestions. They are reserved for a very special situation and intended to be used *only* when working closely with a physician who understands these issues. Most people should do well with a modified Mediterranean-style diet, once they customize it to their individual needs.

Keep your old daily logs, should you ever need to get back on track. Once routine, you will no longer monitor and log every move, but should continue to check A1c periodically and test your glucose on a schedule you and your physician agree upon. It will become a new lifestyle for you. When you have dealt with your diabetes and learned that you have the ability to control it, you have opened the door to a new and healthier lifestyle.

Go and enjoy it.

15

Supplements and Extra Medications

Some diabetics and dieters may need additional nutritional supplements or prescription medication. Others may already be on prescription medication that needs to be reduced or changed as they control their diabetes and lose weight. Earlier, we discussed the need to closely monitor reduce or eliminate your diabetic medication. In this chapter we will focus on additional items.

Anti-hypertensive medication. There's a good chance if you are overweight and diabetic. you are on at least one and often several different pills to control your blood pressure. When you begin this plan, there is no immediate change in your need for these medications. However, as the insulin resistance in your body decreases and you've lost a significant amount of weight, your blood pressure control may improve substantially. Therefore, after a few months or after losing 20 to 30 pounds, your blood pressure medication may be too much. This will become obvious if you suddenly feel faint or dizzy when changing position such as going from sitting to standing. This is called *orthostatic hypotension*. If you take your blood pressure at home, I suggest that you take it in a sitting position and immediately repeat it after standing up. Record these readings. If there is a significant drop when you stand, it is likely that your blood pressure medication needs to be reduced. Your record of these home readings will help your physician decide about medication changes. Usually, people see their physician and have a single blood-pressure reading done in the office. Your physician may be reluctant to reduce your medication based on a single reading, but, if you have been keeping a record over time, the need to change will be obvious. If you are going to be losing a significant amount of weight, be prepared to go through this several times.

Thyroid medication. If you are currently on thyroid medication, this diet should not change your need for it. However, there is a possibility that you may be hypothyroid because you have mistakenly put yourself on a low iodine diet by eliminating iodized table salt. See the section later in this chapter on iodine for more information.

Lithium and blood thinners. I bring up these two different types of medication because these could be sensitive to changes in diet. Since these are medications where exact blood levels are important, be sure that your primary physician keeps a close watch on your blood levels while dieting.

Cholesterol-regulating medications. If you have been started on these medications and are not having any difficulty with them, continue to take them as prescribed. Generally, people on this diet will see an improvement in their overall cholesterol picture. In addition to lower total cholesterol, you may see an increase in your good HDL cholesterol. Combining this with your cholesterol medication may be synergistic. However, a large number of people on statin medications develop muscular pain and weakness. This is often overlooked because when people have not been forewarned, they may not report this to the specialist prescribing the statin medications. If your physician is in a hurry and doesn't remember to ask, it is possible you have been suffering from this for some time.

Some physicians believe that people should be continued on this medication despite their pain and inability to do normal tasks unless blood test shows serious muscular breakdown. However, my belief is that when this problem occurs, action should be taken. One course of action is to immediately start a supplement called Coenzyme Q10, discussed later in this chapter. If this relieves the muscle pain and weakness, it may be possible to continue safely utilizing your cholesterol medication. However, if it does not, you may be extremely sensitive to all statin medications and should not use them. Another possibility is to utilize the vitamin niacin to regulate cholesterol. This can be highly effective but must be used in a specific way discussed later in this chapter.

Vitamin D. Just in the past few years, doctors are learning how little we actually understand about vitamin D. For years, it is been recognized that small amounts of vitamin D were necessary to promote proper bone growth in children when they did not receive enough sunshine. A century ago charities were formed to send children from the slums, where they had little sun exposure, to outdoor summer camps just for the sunlight supplementation. Our bodies actually make our own vitamin D, provided that we have sufficient outdoor activity and sun exposure.

In recent years people around the world have been spending more time indoors because of the comfort of air-conditioning as well as the fear of skin cancer. Now, we realize we may have gone too far. Without sufficient sun exposure, our bodies cannot make enough vitamin D in the summertime to store for use over the winter.

It is now known that vitamin D is more of an internal hormone then a vitamin. Not only is it necessary for bone growth in children, it also is required for maintaining strong bones in adults. In addition, and more importantly, it plays a vital role in regulating our immune system. People with vitamin D deficiencies often have repeated infections or are susceptible to certain dangerous infections. A century ago, before we had drugs to treat tuberculosis, people suffering from this disease were often sent to special hospitals where they were kept in bright sunlight for every daylight hour. Back then, they did not understand the mechanism but understood the relationship between sun exposure and fighting tuberculosis. Recently, studies of the human immune system have shown that vitamin D produced by sunlight, is instrumental in helping the human body fight this particular infection.

Fibromyalgia and myofascial pain syndrome are some recent diseases that can be traced back to vitamin D deficiency. Once rare, these have been increasingly common in the past several years as people receive less sunlight exposure. Although a small amount of vitamin D (often 400 units) is found in most multivitamins, the current thinking is that the daily requirement is probably somewhere between 2000 and 5000 units. Vitamin D may also play a role in depression, particularly when it has a seasonal component.

If you feel that you may have a vitamin D deficiency, ask your physician for a blood test. Healthiest values are in the high normal range. If you require a supplement, the most effective form of vitamin D is D3 or cholecalciferol, which is available inexpensively without a prescription. Discuss this need with your physician. If you have been extremely low, you may require an extra large dose for a short period of time to bring your body up to adequate levels. Diabetics may be at a greater risk for this deficiency than others.

Chapter 15   *Supplements and Extra Medications*

Magnesium. As many as one-fourth of diabetics may have a pre-existing magnesium deficiency. Although some magnesium is found in multivitamin preparations, you may need more. One symptom of a magnesium deficiency is nighttime muscle cramping, particularly in the legs. Some dieters experience this once they begin this diet. This quickly responds to a magnesium supplement. A good combination supplement containing magnesium, calcium, zinc, and a small amount of vitamin D is available without a prescription.

Folate. An important B vitamin is also known as folic acid. Both diabetics and people who are significantly obese tend to be deficient in folate. In the past, folate was best known for its role in preventing anemia. Both a folate deficiency and a vitamin B12 deficiency cause the same type of anemia, characterized by a low blood cell count but swollen, oversize red blood cells.

In a strange twist, dietary supplementation with the vitamin folate had been deliberately restricted in the past. Given enough folate, someone with a vitamin B12 deficiency would not become anemic, so the condition would not be spotted on a routine blood test. A severe B12 deficiency can also cause neurological problems, so it was felt that it was wiser to risk folate deficiency to be able to uncover B12 problems easily.

Today, this thinking has changed for two reasons. Vitamin B12 deficiency can easily be detected by a simple blood test.

This should no longer be excuse for a limiting folate. A number of years ago, it was recognized that low folate levels in pregnant women caused neural tube defects in their children. Since then, folate is more readily available in adequate amounts, particularly in vitamins labeled as "prenatal vitamins." Around the world, governments began to fortify common foods with folate.

More recently, it was found that folate protects against heart disease and reduces hypertension by limiting homocysteine. Taking folate also is associated with a substantially lower risk of developing colon cancer. However, there is controversy about this, because low blood levels of folate levels (as opposed to dietary intake) also seem associated with lower colon cancer rates. Additionally, women who already have colon polyps and take extra folate may experience addition progression of these.

Some dieters may experience hair thinning while dieting. Hair thinning is sometimes caused by inadequate folate, and if this is the case, it may be reversible with adequate doses of folate. Should you experience this problem, prenatal vitamins or a folate supplement may be helpful.

Folate can be found naturally in green leafy vegetables. If you believe you need extra folate, you may want to have your physician check your blood level and provide a recommendation. The usual recommendation is 400 mcg (micrograms) daily but double that in pregnancy. Research in heart disease has sometimes used much higher levels.

Vitamin B12. Vitamin B12 is important for both blood forming and the nervous system. Multivitamins contain adequate amounts for most people. Deficiencies are usually found only in people who avoid red meat and do not take vitamin supplements. There is a condition where vitamin B12 cannot be absorbed in adequate amounts and must be given in the form of a monthly injection. After having stomach surgery, particularly gastric bypass, deficiency of vitamin B12 is common. If you have previously undergone such surgery, you should be tested for vitamin B12 deficiency and started on regular injections.

Chromium. This trace mineral is a cofactor in maintaining glucose control. Although a lack of chromium has be shown to be a factor for developing diabetes in an animal model, it is not clear whether this is an important consideration in people. Some research scientists advocate its use, in amounts of 1,000 mcg (micrograms) each day. Small amounts are available in some multivitamins. It is found in pharmacies and health food stores as Chromium Picolinate.

Carnitine. Carnitine is needed to burn fat. Although most people probably receive an adequate supply in their diet, people who avoid red meat may be deficient. Those vegetarians who avoid all animal products are most likely to be deficient. If you have difficulty initiating and maintaining fat burning, you might benefit from this supplement. It is sold in pharmacies and health food stores as L-Carnitine. You may need to take 1,000 to 2,000 mg or more each day.

DHEA. Dehydroepiandrosterone is normally made within the body. It is turned into sex hormones. Many exaggerated claims have been made by those profiting from its sale. Research has shown that it may be useful in decreasing abdominal fat, but should be used cautiously.

Taking it <u>may</u> help the body increase its level of testosterone in both men and women. This <u>may</u> increase energy level and sex drive while decreasing depression, but it has drawbacks. People suffering from polycystic ovary disorder, heart disease, or surviving any form of cancer that is sensitive to hormones would be wise to avoid using this.

Niacin. Niacin is an important B vitamin. In developed countries, most people get enough niacin in their diet to prevent niacin deficiency. However, in larger doses and in the right form, niacin has a useful function in improving cholesterol balance. Correctly used, it is inexpensive, available without a prescription and more effective than the riskier statin drugs. In addition, it is sometimes used in conjunction with statin drugs for a powerful combination. Although its superiority has been well understood for about four decades, the fact that it is not patentable means that you will not see it in those expensive television commercials, the ones being used to get people on more costly medication. **Niacin not only lowers bad cholesterol, it simultaneously increases HDL good cholesterol!**

If your physician wants to improve your cholesterol balanced, this is an excellent addition to the improvements you should already be getting from following the plan. If you have been on a statin drug and developed muscle pain or weakness, this is an excellent source. People who should not take niacin include pregnant women and anyone with liver disease.

Two problems with niacin are either that people buy it in the wrong form or they take it wrong way. Niacin comes in three forms. Only the form called nicotinic acid has the cholesterol-lowering effect. The other forms of niacin will prevent pellagra or niacin deficiency but nothing more. These other forms are niacinamide and inositol hexaniotinate. Plain niacin, in the form of nicotinic acid, is very inexpensive. Expect to pay about 5¢ a pill. Look for the container to either clearly state that it is nicotinic acid or contain a warning about expecting a flush. Never buy a flush-free niacin. It is a waste of money that is being marketed falsely, since it typically contains inositol hexaniotinate. Niacinamide, the type of niacin found in multivitamins will not help lower your cholesterol either.

The drawback of nicotinic acid is that shortly after it is taken blood vessels in your skin will open causing a red flush accompanied by a sensation of burning and itching. This may last for several minutes. Many people have simply bought niacin without following the proper protocol, encountered the flushing and never tried it again.

When starting niacin, it is important to find the smallest size that you can, typically 250 or 500 mg, breaking it into quarters and start on this small daily dose. Take an aspirin shortly before taking the niacin. A small 81 mg baby aspirin or cardiac aspirin is perfect. You should barely feel the flush and after doing this for several days, increase to a half-tablet for a few more days as your body becomes accustomed to niacin. Gradually work your way up until you are taking several pills a day for a total of 1500 to 2000 mg. Doing it this way, you should find the flushing to be tolerable and barely noticeable.

In an effort to reduce the flushing, several formulations of slow-release niacin have come on the market, both in prescription and non-prescription forms. Although this seemed like a good idea, it turns out that slow-release niacin can be extremely irritating to your liver. Be sure that your physician knows you are taking niacin and checks your liver as part of your annual blood chemistry.

Co-enzyme Q10. Taking a co-enzyme Q10 supplement is normally not needed. However, if you have been started on any statin drug it is very important. A statin drug may rob your body this important coenzyme and lead to muscular problems. If you take a statin drug, consider this supplement.

Iodine.   The mineral iodine is important for human life. In the past, natural dietary intake of iodine varied by where you lived. Living near a seacoast and consuming fresh fish was helpful in maintaining adequate levels of iodine. In the 1920s the disease of hypothyroidism caused by a lack of iodine was recognized as plaguing many people living in the Midwestern United States. The addition of potassium iodide to ordinary table salt largely corrected this problem. This simple solution worked so well that its purpose has been largely forgotten.

Today, once again, large numbers of people suffer from iodine deficiency, which should become evident when they are diagnosed with hypothyroidism. Unfortunately, properly testing for iodine deficiency requires a 24-hour urine collection, making the test cumbersome and expensive. It is rarely tested for today. Instead people with hypothyroidism are simply placed on prescription thyroid hormone.

Why has this happened? For three decades the government has been critical of salt consumption in the American diet. This imbalance of dietary sodium has been blamed on ordinary salt because the food industry has diverted attention away from the fact that almost all processed foods contain monosodium glutamate, often hidden in innocent sounding "broths." Many people listened to this message and eliminated table salt from their diet. This has completely undone the effort to have adequate an dietary intake of iodine.

Curiously, the United States contributes money to the World Health Organization so that nations of Africa will switch to the use of iodized salt to prevent hypothyroidism. This has decreased the subsequent problem of iodine deficiency in pregnant women causing their children to be born with neurologic deficits. Despite giving this advice to other nations, at home the confused message about sodium has caused many people to eliminate all iodized table salt from their daily diet.

Dietary iodine is necessary for normal thyroid gland function. When you are following this plan, you are avoiding all the processed foods containing hidden sodium. Adequate use of iodized table salt will provide you with extra iodine you may be lacking. If you have been diagnosed with hypothyroidism, discuss the possibility of testing your iodine level with your physician. Take a potassium iodide supplement, if it is indicated by this test.

Metabolism boosters. Avoid all products claiming to boost your metabolism to lose weight. These are all variants on a theme and all pose the same dangers. Over-the-counter products change their formulations one step ahead of government regulators. Prescription formulations come on the market claiming complete safety, only to be severely restricted or pulled off the market several years later, after damaging or killing people.

This is not a new development. In the 1890s cocaine was a popular weight-loss prescription. Beginning in the 1930's, so was amphetamine!

There may be other supplements that you will hear about. Be cautious and trust your physician before trusting claims made by people or companies trying to sell you their product.

16

Protecting Others

There is ancient religious dictum that states *"If you save one life it is as if you have saved the entire world."* If every person in the world were able to save just one life, it would change the entire world. At the beginning of this book I explained the magnitude of the diabetes and obesity epidemics. This combination is changing the entire world. How can you, simply one person, expect to change the world? The answer is that you begin one person at a time.

Begin with yourself. As you become successful in controlling and reversing your diabetes, you will become an example for those around you. Family members who are not yet diabetic and were reluctant to admit their own need for weight-loss can suddenly become interested. Your example can lead them to save their own lives. These dual epidemics of obesity and diabetes are killing people. Anyone you have encouraged by your example can be a life that will be saved.

You may not think of yourself as a crusader or leader on a campaign to save the world, but what about your own family? You do not have to pressure anyone. Leading by example is one of the most powerful statements that you can make. If there are other members of your family who need help, your success can be the light that guides them. I have seen this time and again when someone who is successfully reversing diabetes and losing weight announces that his or her spouse decided to follow them and is being equally successful.

When you lead by example, you do not have to be confrontational. You do not have to tell others that they need to diet or change their lifestyle. You know from your own experience how unpleasant that can be. People who are overweight know they need to diet but do not believe that they can succeed. Diabetics who are poorly controlled are often trying to follow the advice they had been given and have been falsely blamed by their dietician or physician for not trying hard enough. Your example can give them hope, just as a friend's success may have given you hope. Your success can be infectious. When you are successful at it, other people in your group will focus on what you did and copy you.

This is the first way you are protecting your family and others around you. Those who are already in trouble will benefit from your example. There is a second important way that you can protect those you love. Although your children may not need to lose weight or control their blood sugar yet, they might be started on the same path you had followed. The knowledge that you have acquired following your plan will serve them well.

No, those who are not yet overweight do not need to diet nor should they be in ketosis. Instead, they need to avoid the pitfalls that could lead to their impaired glucose tolerance and obesity. You have the power to influence them and keep them off the path to diabetes.

You can start by getting the junk food out of your house. By this time, you should have an understanding of what I mean by junk food. Start with beverages. Water is the best drink you can find in your home. If your municipal water supply has problems with taste or odor, get a filter. Even a simple filter pitcher works well. If your family has become addicted to sweet-tasting soft drinks, wean them gradually. Eliminate the sugar kick that they get by switching to diet soda. Have your children drink water with their school lunch, not those little juice boxes. Make sure that candies and cakes are treats, reserved for holidays and special occasions.

Use pure meats at your table, not the broth-injected type. Stay away from ready-to-eat meals that you take from the freezer and put into the microwave. Avoid MSG in all their foods. Be especially wary of canned or powdered soups. Avoid those tasty MSG-laden cans of spaghetti and ravioli aimed at youngsters. Make their breakfast more wholesome by eliminating flavored cereals and toaster pastries. Most varieties of those breakfast foods are loaded with sugar. Use real dairy products in your home, not the imitation substitutes.

You will meet less resistance to these moves than you anticipate. If your family has seen you undergo a remarkable change through your plan, they will have a better understanding when you explain why you are taking certain steps.

Those you love are not with you twenty-four hours each day. When your loved ones are away at school or work, they are in a totally different atmosphere. As you make changes at home, educate them as to why you are doing these things. Let them know what they need to avoid outside of the home. Consider packing lunches for them so that they can avoid those school lunches, which are now under the thumb of the food industry.

Once you have your family on your side, look for other places that limit your healthy choices. Think about the potluck dinners at your church or synagogue. Suggest healthier dishes to others there. Do not be a pest about it, but explain that these are steps that helped you get slim and are helping protect your family. If the community around you has seen you get healthier, they will respect what you have to say.

If you have children in school, make yourself heard in your school system. School superintendents and school boards are local. They listen to parents who stand up for what is right. Do not tackle the issues under state and federal control yet. You will learn how the food lobby has many state and federal regulators under their thumb. This makes it difficult for local school boards to exert independence in some aspects. As an example, you might have local farmers who would be thrilled to be able to sell fresh produce to your school. Instead, the school often must buy from major food companies, shipping from thousand of miles away, because of blanket contracts and restrictions from the state.

Instead, go after shady local practices that can be controlled. Even in small communities, local school boards can be enticed by fees running into hundreds of thousands of dollars from the soft drink industry. They pay these fees to put soda machines in the schools, replacing water fountains for thirsty youngsters. Go back to water. When school budgets are tight, dangling these huge amounts in front of school superintendents trying to balance their budgets is extremely enticing. Put your foot down. Soft drink vending machines have no place in public schools. These are your children that these companies are trying to entice. Would you let a crack dealer set up shop with in the halls of your schools if he gave the school board $200,000? Of course not. Yet, soft drink companies get into bidding wars to get their brands into our school systems.

Know your enemy. The battle for good food has many enemies. Some are benign in their intent but do much harm from their ignorance. Others are highly malevolent and knowingly put their business interests ahead of the public good. Many are multi-national players, who could care less about the health of individuals in your community. Some of them play dirty. The boxes that follow on the next few pages contain problems explaining how these companies play dirty and why our government is inept at fighting them. Study them and be wary. If you go beyond the local level, to your state and federal legislatures, expect to see these tactics at work.

Do not be discouraged. By starting with yourself and your family, you have a solid foundation. Working from that you can change your community.

The nine boxes that follow show some of the problems that now exist. Understanding these problems will help you fight for a safer food supply. Eventually, we may have truly pure foods and honest truth-in-labeling, but only if people like you work for it!

If you save one life,
it is as if you have saved the entire world.

Problem 1

Weakened Safety Enforcement

The original *Pure Food and Drug Act* was passed more than a century ago. It brought about radical improvement in the trust we could give to the food industry. Over the years, the effectiveness of food regulation has been eroded as lawyers for the food processors have figured out end runs against regulation after regulation. The cozy relationship of the regulators with the regulated has worsened this problem.

Until the government looks at every single food additive and demands safety testing at least as rigorous as they do for medication, we must treat the safety of food additives with great skepticism. Until the government demands clear and unequivocal labeling of food ingredients, we must be wary of anything we eat.

Problem 2

Organized Malevolence

If you have read about the malevolent acts the tobacco industry was infamous for in the past, would it surprise you that the food processing industry they now control is following the same playbook? Just as the tobacco industry spent many millions of dollars setting up phony institutes and foundations to plead their cause, so has the food industry.

Organizations exist with high-sounding names to tell us all about food safety. These organizations are funded by the food industry. Is it any wonder that they continually whitewash and distort the truth about the dangers of food additives, faux foods, and the resultant obesity epidemic!

By appearing to be concerned about the public good, these organizations can reassure naive individuals who are concerned about food issues. Do not be one of them! You can see by your own success in avoiding these faux foods that there are real issues concerning our food supply.

Problem 3

Muffling the Truth

Right now, there is a tremendous effort to muffle the truth about pure products. There is a chemical called bovine growth hormone or BGH that is given to dairy cows to increase their milk production. Many small dairy farmers would rather produce a pure product. These small dairies have been letting the public know that their dairy herds are not being given BGH. The producer of BGH fears that this will make the public aware of the practice that many large dairies use.

To stop this threat to their chemical sale, a tremendous lobbying effort is underway in state legislatures across the nation to pass laws to silence these small dairies. If passed, dairies selling chemically free milk would be banned from saying this. Even worse, the legislation drafted by the chemical company essentially bans informing the public if any product is free of anything. This legislation passed recently in the state of Pennsylvania. Fortunately, when the public became aware of this bill, public outrage caused the governor to veto it. That has not stopped the chemical producers from introducing the same restrictions in other states.

BGH is not an issue in this diet but silencing and distorting truth is. This example demonstrates how with enough money, enough lobbying and enough lawyers, the truth about food products can be withheld from the public.

Problem 4

Lack of Federal Health Leadership

Virtually any nation you can think of has a Secretary or Minister of Health—a cabinet position leading a government department, taking responsibility for the health of that nation. This occurs in virtually any nation you can think of—except for the United States of America.

We have never had a Secretary of Health. Instead, we have had a Secretary of Health and something. Health, Education, and Welfare; Health and Human Services, and so forth. We totally lack health leadership at a level that even most third-world countries enjoy. Instead, we have a lot of small, compartmentalized government departments marching to different drummers. Sometimes they have no responsibility in a particular area. At other times, they have conflicting responsibility.

Yes, we have a Surgeon General. Yet, this person is a figurehead who has no authority to command our various health bureaucracies. The Surgeon General is the ranking officer of the Public Health Commissioned Corps, a leftover from the days of sailing ships where a naval medical officer boarded ships arriving in our harbor to determine whether they had to be quarantined. That is why the Surgeon General is seen in a naval outfit. Many employees in the federal health bureaucracy are members of this Commissioned Corps, allowing them to receive benefits that equal those of military officers. The

continued on next page

Problem 4 continued

Surgeon General does not command them in their daily activities. Instead, they report to whatever branch of the bureaucracy they are assigned.

The Surgeon General is always a physician, although quite a few have been physicians who had no qualifications or training in public health. This political appointee sits at a level many layers below the Secretary of Health and Human Services in the organizational chart.

Is it any wonder that the federal government's efforts to preserve our health often go astray?

Problem 5

Handcuffed State Health Leadership

Once, individual state health departments provided important leadership in this country. Today, health leadership within states varies widely. Although state health departments often have tremendous legal authority to protect their citizens, the federal government has handcuffed them.

Restricted federal funds form a significant share of a state health department's budget. All the other things that they would like to do receive little money. For practical purposes, most state health departments find their hands tied when they want to speak out about something that is not a federal priority.

Food companies take advantage of this weakness. Whenever food companies see a state take the initiative in health matters, they argue the case for federal jurisdiction. An example is when states want to give additional package information or otherwise restrict a product. Food companies can spend tremendous amounts to hire sophisticated legal teams and tie the issue up in court for years. Few states feel they have the resources to battle this issue in court.

Problem 6

Whitewashing Dangerous Problems

The food industry knows that a consumer revolt can be a powerful force to initiate effective regulation. Therefore, they have embarked on a misinformation campaign, designed to placate the public into believing that there are no dangers from food additives.

One method that they use to do this is to plant articles in well-read magazines and newspapers that imply that these additives are both natural and harmless. As an example, when you see a food article that talks about dangerous additives as *"not having been conclusively proven to do any harm except in sensitive individuals"* that is lawyer-speak. It is intended to confuse you into believing that a substance was proven harmless. In fact, many of these additives entered our food chain without any form of testing. Others have been tested by antiquated standards that were originally intended only to keep substances such as arsenic out of our food.

This does not stop these planted pieces from appearing in important and well-read publications. They are a product of a well thought out public relations campaigns on the part of the food processing and chemical industry. They are appearing more often today, as the food industry recognizes their precarious position.

This tactic is straight from the tobacco industry playbook, from when they denied cigarettes did harm!

Problem 7

Immunity from Lawsuits.

Food companies know that trial lawyers filing multi-billion dollar class action suits can be powerful adversaries. These aggressive lawyers have helped to rein in some of the nastier things in our society. It is far easier for the powerful food companies to squelch effective laws and regulation than it is to stop trial lawyers who believe they have a good case against companies with lots of money.

Although the Constitution of the United States gives citizens the right to sue when harmed, the food processing lobby would like to be above that. They think that they deserve the type of sovereign immunity given to ancient kings. They have attempted to get such immunity any way they can.

One way was to attempt to pass a federal law that would exempt food producers and purveyors from responsibility for obesity. Fortunately, this ridiculous law did not pass the U.S. Congress. However, they have been successful in another way.

A few years ago, a group of attorneys sued all the MSG producers for price-fixing. They did not sue on behalf of the food manufacturers who paid for the MSG in their packaged foods. Instead, they sued on behalf of all consumers in the United States. The theory of their suit was that the increased price of MSG led to an increased price in processed foods and so consumers should

continued on next page

receive the benefit of this. Of course, they could not get the individual consumers, every individual living in the United States, to sign on to this. Instead, they went to the attorneys general of all of the individual states. They promised them that instead of awarding a few pennies to each individual, their state treasuries would get the money they were able to win. About three-fourths of the states agreed to this supposed windfall.

Subsequently, they drew up a negotiated agreement with the MSG producers. That agreement had these producers pay a relatively small amount of money, which was to be split up among the state treasuries and the lawyers.

The court allowed them to post a small, incomprehensible notice in national magazines telling people that they would be a party to lawsuits unless they notified the court that they were opting out of it. Therefore, any citizen who did not send a letter to the court was automatically included as a plaintiff and went along with the negotiated settlement agreed to by these attorneys. Their proposed settlement stated that *you could never sue the MSG companies for anything else*, not just things related to the supposed MSG price-fixing.

Fortunately, the court did not approve this tricky language and it was deleted from the settlement the court did approve. Nice try! Would a trial attorney have tried to sue an MSG maker on behalf of anyone unknowingly included in that proposed settlement? Was this a tricky way to try to gain immunity from lawsuits for the physical harm done to innocent people? What do you think?

Problem 8

Stacking the Deck

Today, responsibility for food safety is split among government agencies, primarily the Food and Drug Administration (FDA) and the Department of Agriculture (USDA). Recent events have shown that these agencies may not get out into the field to inspect the processors they are supposedly regulating. In addition, they accept food companies at their word, even when the food processors buy chemicals from faceless foreign suppliers.

Food safety has always been a poor stepchild at the FDA. Many additives have been deemed safe simply because they have been around for many years. The food processing industry is happy to draft the regulations for them and tell them what to do. When the FDA needs expert advice about a food additive, to whom do they turn: people with numerous financial ties to the food industry, scientists who provide consultation to the food processors, and universities with contracts from these same food companies.

Problem 9

Food and Drugs have Blended

Today, there is no clear line between the mega-companies that manufacture and control seemingly unrelated products. The agricultural and chemical companies work together to create genetically modified products, whether plants or animals. When drug companies do not have the effectiveness data to receive government approval for a new drug, they may find a way to market it as a nutritional substance. When food manufactures need a new artificial ingredient, they may turn to a drug company to develop it.

Combine this with the multi-billion dollar profits currently being made by both the pharmaceutical and food industries due to the epidemics of diabetes, obesity, and resultant diseases.

The astronomical profits involved provide a powerful incentive for corner-cutting, half-truths, and manipulation. This is not the place for *laissez-faire* deregulation, such as we saw in the oil industry debacle.

Understanding these major problems will not solve them, but it is a first step in fighting them.

17

Meal Plans and Recipes

This chapter offers practical meal plans and recipes for starting your diet. As you become accustomed to the 60-40-10 plan, you will find yourself varying what you eat and becoming more creative. However, many people asked me for a practical starting plan, which this represents. As you review the meal plans, remember their use is optional. If there are foods you cannot or will not eat on a particular day, skip them. Substitute the menu for another day or another meal.

The first section includes meal plans for a full week. Some of the food items are special recipes found at the beginning of the recipe section that follows. These meal plans are a starting point and only approximate the 60-40-10 plan. As you select menu items from them, you will still need to use your daily log to check your totals. Each recipe is in a format giving approximate nutritional totals, There are additional recipes for you to use that are not in the first seven days of the meal plan.

Many additional recipes will be found in *Cooking for the New Hippocratic Diet™, ISBN 978-0-9820111-7-1,* soon to be available at bookstores or www.HippocraticDiet.com.

Newer recipes are at posted at www.HippocraticDiet.com and change periodically. Some recipes are ones we developed while others have been developed and submitted by users of this plan. Some of these submitted recipes were based upon older recipes, which they adapted to the requirements of this diet. I am grateful to all those who have submitted recipes.

If you have the time, you should recheck recipes that you use, since error values can vary with different brands of ingredients. Because of such differences as well as variations in cooking methods, all nutritional values should be treated as estimates and exact values may vary.

Calculations for nutritional analysis has been largely based upon ingredient data. In this, we used either accepted data, government–provided data or manufacturer-provided data. Unfortunately, this has limitations. This is particularly true in the United States, where manufacturers have significant legal leeway in presenting factual data. We try to note where we have questions. Should any recipe seem to cause an unexpected rise in blood sugar or reduction in ketosis, please inform us through our website www.HippocraticDiet.com.

Be especially wary of low-carbohydrate recipes found on the Internet. Although there are useful recipes to be found, many contain serious errors. Some supposedly low-carb recipes from the Internet could interrupt both your diabetes recovery and your weight-loss progress.

Following the recipe section, there are planning sheets for you to use to analyze other recipes that you may find or to create your own recipes. If you develop recipes you enjoy, share them with others. I invite you to submit them at www.HippocraticDiet.com for such sharing and possible inclusion in future editions.

Monday

Breakfast

- Coffee with real cream and non-calorie sweetener
- One fluffy egg omelet *(see recipe)*
- One thick *(or 2 regular)* strip*(s)* sugar-free bacon

Lunch

- Small lettuce salad with two grape tomatoes
- Shredded cheese
- Olive oil dressing
- Water or diet soda

Dinner

- Three-to-four ounce steak
- Broccoli with melted cheese
- Water or diet soda

Optional snack

- One-half ounce cashews

Tuesday

Breakfast

- Coffee with real cream and non-calorie sweetener
- One fried egg
- One MSG-free sausage patty

Lunch

- Small lettuce salad with two grape tomatoes
- Sliced cooked chicken *(about an ounce)*
- Bleu cheese dressing *(see recipe)*
- Water or diet soda

Dinner

- Three to four ounce salmon portion
- Small lettuce salad with two grape tomatoes, shredded cheese and olive oil dressing
- Water or diet soda

Optional snack

- One ounce of cheese cubes

Wednesday

Breakfast

- Homemade hot chocolate *(see recipe)*
- One scrambled egg
- One MSG-free sausage link

Lunch

- MSG-free tuna salad on a bed of lettuce
- "Free lemonade" *(see recipe),* water, or diet soda

Dinner

- Three to four ounce pork chop with optional homemade barbecue sauce *(see recipe)*
- Small lettuce salad with two grape tomatoes, shredded cheese, and bleu cheese dressing *(see recipe)*
- Water or diet soda

Optional snack

- One-half ounce almonds

Thursday

Breakfast

- Coffee with real cream and non-calorie sweetener
- One scrambled egg mixed with one ounce cooked or smoked salmon

Lunch

- Small portion mixed greens topped with smoked kippers
- Olive oil dressing
- Water or diet soda

Dinner

- Hearty chicken stew *(see recipe)*
- Small lettuce salad with two grape tomatoes, shredded cheese, and olive oil dressing
- Water or diet soda

Optional snack

- One ounce olives

Friday

Breakfast

- Coffee with real cream and non-calorie sweetener
- One fluffy egg omelet *(see recipe)*
- One thick *(or 2 regular)* strip*(s)* sugar-free bacon

Lunch

- Small lettuce salad with two grape tomatoes
- Sliced cooked chicken *(about an ounce)*
- Bleu cheese dressing *(see recipe)*
- Water or diet soda

Dinner

- Three-to-four ounces chicken topped with homemade mole sauce *(see recipe)*
- Small lettuce salad with and olive oil dressing
- Water or diet soda

Optional snack

- Sugar-free Jell-O™ topped with homemade whipped cream *(see recipe)*

Saturday

Breakfast

- Coffee with real cream and non-calorie sweetener
- One scrambled egg
- One thick *(or 2 regular)* strip*(s)* sugar-free bacon

Lunch

- Small lettuce salad with two grape tomatoes
- Sliced cooked chicken *(about an ounce)*
- Bleu cheese dressing *(see recipe)*
- Water or diet soda

Dinner

- Four ounce portion lamb breast
- Lightly steamed asparagus with creamy curry sauce *(see recipe)*
- Water or diet soda

Optional snack

- Real cream soda *(see recipe)*

Sunday

Breakfast

- Coffee with real cream and non-calorie sweetener
- One fluffy egg omelet *(see recipe)*
- One MSG-free sausage link

Lunch

- Small lettuce salad topped with sesame oil
- Hearty chicken stew *(see recipe)*
- Water or diet soda

Dinner

- Three-to-four ounce portion of salmon
- Small lettuce salad with two grape tomatoes, shredded cheese, and feta cheese dressing *(see recipe)*
- Water or diet soda

Optional snack

- One ounce olives

Fluffy Egg Omelet

Nutritionally, this is the same as an omelet made in the normal way but once you try it, you will appreciate its flavor, texture, and size. Using a single egg, it provides about the same size portion as an ordinary two egg omelet. If you are not used to separating eggs, buy a simple egg separator at a kitchen or housewares store.

Ingredients	Amount
Large egg	1
Heavy cream	1 teaspoon
Extra-virgin olive oil (or butter)	1 teaspoon
Salt, pepper, or spice	to taste

Instructions: Separate the egg white from the yolk. Using an electric mixer or a hand whisk, beat the egg white until it is very frothy and increased in volume. Heat the olive oil (or butter) in a frying pan. Lightly blend the egg yolk and spices into the frothy egg white. Pour the mixture into the heated frying pan. Cook until done, flipping or covering to be sure that the top is done.

If you are cooking for several people, be sure to use a large pan. This recipe produces a thick, fluffy omelet. The air you whisked in will insulate the top of the omelet from the cooking heat unless you use a large pan to allow the mixture to spread out.

Energy	**127 calories**
Fat	**11 grams**
Protein	**6 grams**
Carbohydrate	**1 gram**

Chunky Bleu or Feta Cheese Dressing

Use this as a salad dressing, a sauce to top meat, fish and vegetables or as a dip for celery.

Ingredients	Amount
Crumpled bleu cheese or feta cheese	¼ cup
Real mayonnaise	½ cup
Real sour cream	1 cup
Hot sauce *(optional)*	A few drops, to taste

Instructions: Mix ingredients. Refrigerate unused portion.

Serving Size: About 2 tablespoons

Energy	**62 calories**
Fat	**6 grams**
Protein	**1 grams**
Carbohydrate	**1 gram**

Hot Chocolate

Use this recipe when you need a chocolate lift or to warm yourself on a dreary winter day. You also may refrigerate it to serve cold, either by itself or mixed with club soda.

Ingredients	Amount
100% cocoa powder	1 teaspoon
Heavy cream	1 tablespoon
Non-calorie sweetener	to taste
Hot water	to fill cup

Instructions: Pour hot to boiling water over cocoa powder and stir until dissolved. Add cream, sweeten to taste and stir.

Energy	**65 calories**
Fat	**5 ½ grams**
Protein	**1 gram**
Carbohydrate	**3 grams**

Diabetes Recovery

Free Lemonade

This is a strategy to cope with problems when eating out, but it also works at home. When eating out, the only non-calorie beverage choices are often either water or something containing caffeine. If you do not want to have caffeine with your meal, too bad. Here is a way to fight back. It is free of both sugar and caffeine, as well as free-of-charge.

Ingredients	Amount
Water	1 glass
Lemon	1 slice
Non-calorie sweetener	to taste

Instructions: When eating out, ask for a slice of lemon in your water. Squeeze the lemon into you glass and use non-calorie sweetener to taste. If you tip the waitress a little more for her trouble, you still save money compared to a soft drink. At home, try using concentrated lemon or lime juice.

Energy	**0 calories**
Fat	**0 grams**
Protein	**0 grams**
Carbohydrate	**0 grams**

Barbecue and Meat Sauce

This is a terrific sauce for cooking meat and as a base for other sauces. It is calorie-free and can be made up in advance and stored. The key ingredient is chipotle sauce, a thick brown sauce made from smoked chili peppers. It can be found in the Mexican food section of many supermarkets and specialty stores.

<u>Ingredients</u>	<u>Amount</u>
Chipotle sauce *(additive-free)*	All quantities to taste
Ground cinnamon	All quantities to taste
Non-calorie liquid sweetener	All quantities to taste
Fresh or bottled lemon juice	All quantities to taste

Instructions: Mix ingredients together until completely blended. Quantities can be varied to your taste. Brush on meat or chicken before cooking.

Energy	**0 calories**
Fat	**0 grams**
Protein	**0 grams**
Carbohydrate	**0 grams**

Chicken Mole

Mole, pronounced *mo-lay*, is a Mexican dish which has many regional variations. They contain chocolate, ground nuts, chili pepper, other spices and sweetener. This recipe does not claim authenticity but it is tasty. Vary it as you like. It works well with other dishes besides chicken, too.

Ingredients:	*Amount:*
Chicken breast	½ portion, about 4 oz.
Olive oil	2 tablespoons
100% cocoa powder	1 teaspoon
Cinnamon	½ teaspoon, to taste
Liquid non-calorie sweetener	1 teaspoon, to taste
Hot pepper sauce	½ teaspoon, to taste
Natural peanut butter	1 teaspoon, to taste
Ground red pepper	½ teaspoon, to taste

Instructions: Cook chicken by sautéing it in oil in a frying pan. Lower heat to simmer and mix in the other ingredients. Stir to mix as peanut butter softens. Add a little water or MSG-free chicken broth to thin, if needed. Cover and simmer for a few minutes to allow flavors to mix. Add other ingredients, such as sliced mushrooms if desired. You may also want to try this as a meat or chicken stir-fry, featuring cut-up leftovers and vegetables.

Energy	178	calories
Fat	18	grams
Protein	27	grams
Carbohydrate	2 net carbs	grams

Hearty Chicken Stew

This is too thick and rich to call chicken soup. Stew is a much better description for this hearty main course. It bears no resemblance to those MSG-laden canned broths, but might resemble something recognizable by your great-grandparents.

Ingredients (for 4 servings)	Amount
Chicken leg quarter	1 (about 1 lb)
Water	10 cups
Celery	2 stalks
Carrots	2
Old Bay Seasoning ™ or celery salt or celery seed	to taste
Salt and pepper	to taste
Onion (optional)	to taste
Mushroom stems and pieces (optional)	1 small (4 oz) can or use fresh mushrooms

Instructions: Use a large pot or an electric crock-pot or slow cooker. Remove any attached organs from the chicken but leave the skin and fat on. Cut the celery and carrots into about ½ inch long pieces. Place all ingredients but the mushrooms into the pot and bring it to a boil. Reduce heat to a simmer and cover loosely. Allow to simmer several hours. If you are using a crock-pot, it is fine to leave it all day or overnight on a low setting. Cook until the meat is literally falling off the bones. Allow to cool enough to safely handle. Use a strainer, colander or ladle to separate the solids from the broth and then carefully pick out and discard all the bones. Take out all the skin and fat and about half of the meat, place it in an electric blender or food

continued on the next page

processor and purée it. Return all ingredients to the pot, add the mushrooms, bring it back to a boil and let it cook, uncovered until you are ready to serve. For a thick and hearty stew, this should reduce to a volume of about 4 cups.

If you want to serve this as a lighter soup, begin with more water or do not reduce it quite as much. You may also want to save some of the clear broth as a base for other recipes, which call for MSG-free chicken broth.

Hint: For good taste, best results and fewest chemicals, buy a chicken marked "Air-Chilled" or one that does not show any percentage of retained water or broth.

Energy *(per serving)*	**257**	**calories**
Fat	**17**	**grams**
Protein	**20**	**grams**
Carbohydrate	**5**	**grams**

Real Whipped Cream

Many people have forgotten what real whipped cream is. Once you try this, you will never go back to the artificial stuff. Have it plain or on Sugar-Free Jell-O.™

<u>*Ingredients*</u>	<u>**Amount**</u>
Heavy whipping cream	2 tablespoons
Liquid artificial sweetener	To taste

Instructions: Place cream and sweetener in a cool, deep bowl. Using an electric mixer with cool beaters, whip it until it doubles in size and thickens. Store any unused amounts in a closed refrigerator container.

	<u>Alone</u>	<u>With Jell-O™</u>
Energy	90 calories	94 calories
Fat	10 grams	10 grams
Protein	0 grams	1 gram
Carbohydrate	0 grams	0 grams

Note: Use the Sugar-Free Jell-O™ or equivalent that you mix yourself. The pre-mixed cups have added carbohydrates. Use flavors that are marked "5 calories" or less.

Creamy Curry Sauce

This simple sauce is a great way to balance the proportion of fat in meals, while adding taste. It goes with many foods. Try it on lightly steamed asparagus.

Ingredients	Amount
Real Mayonnaise	1 tablespoon
Curry Powder	about ½ teaspoon, to taste

Instructions: Mix the curry powder and mayonnaise thoroughly. Allow to stand a few minutes before using. If larger amounts are mixed, be sure to refrigerate.

Energy	**99 calories**
Fat	**11 grams**
Protein	**0 grams**
Carbohydrate	**0 grams**

Real Cream Soda

Whether you want to increase the proportion of fat in a particular meal or just have a delicious beverage, try this real cream soda.

Ingredients	*Amount*
Diet soda in a flavor such as cola, cream, or root beer	Enough to fill a glass
Heavy cream	1 tablespoon
Ice cubes	

Instructions: Place ice in the glass first, then add the cream. Next, pour in the soda. Stir briefly as it froths. Drink up and enjoy.

Hint:: Works well with most flavors except lemon-flavored.

Energy	**45 calories**
Fat	**5 grams**
Protein	**0 grams**
Carbohydrate	**0 grams**

Diabetes Recovery

Creamy Chocolate Dessert

This simple recipe provides a proportioned balance of energy, while allowing you to feel smug about having a chocolate treat. It is a great addition to a light meal.

Ingredients	*Amount*
Real sour cream	2 tablespoons
100% pure cocoa powder	1 teaspoon
Non-calorie liquid sweetener	to taste

Instructions: Stir together until the chocolate is evenly distributed. Taste and stir in extra sweetener, as needed.

Energy	**65**	**calories**
Fat	**5**	**grams**
Protein	**1**	**grams**
Carbohydrate	**4**	**grams**

Denver Omelet

This uses the recipe for the basic Fluffy Egg Omelet to create a Denver Omelet. The Denver Omelet was first created by Greek immigrant restaurant owners in Denver, giving it a distinct Mediterranean heritage.

<u>Ingredients for basic omelet</u>	<u>Amount</u>
Large egg	1
Heavy cream	1 teaspoon
Extra-virgin olive oil	1 teaspoon
Salt, pepper or spice	to taste

<u>Added ingredients</u>	
Chopped bell peppers (red, green, or mixed)	1 oz
Chopped onions	1 oz
Diced cooked ham or crumbled cooked bacon or sausage	1 oz
Hot pepper sauce	to taste

Instructions: Lightly brown the added ingredients in olive oil in the frying pan, then follow the basic Fluffy Egg Omelet recipe *(page 228)* to mix the basic ingredients and slowly stir in the egg mixture. Allow to brown on one side, then, finish by turning it over to brown on the other side. Allow additional time for thicker mixtures when using the fluffy egg recipe.

Energy	**127**	**calories**
Fat	**14**	**grams**
Protein	**14**	**grams**
Carbohydrate	**7**	**grams**

The extra ingredients increase the protein and carbohydrate of the basic omelet.

Grilled Avocado

Avocados are high in healthy monounsaturated fat. Much of the carbohydrate they contain is in the form of fiber. Tajin,™ a powdered Mexican spice, is MSG-free and contains chili peppers, dehydrated lime and salt. You may wish to add a small amount of tomato sauce or salsa to the avocado when serving.

Instructions: Slice the avocado in half and remove the seed.

Ingredients	_Amount_
Avocado	1/2 per portion
Olive Oil	1 teaspoon
Lemon or lime juice	1 teaspoon
Tajin™ or salt and pepper	to taste

Sprinkle oil, juice, and spice in cavity. Place on hot grill cut side up, heat a few minutes and serve. You may also want try cooking this in a frying pan or under a broiler.

Energy	177	calories
Fat	17	grams
Protein	4	grams
Carbohydrate	2 *net carbs**	grams

* net carbs are explained in Going Shopping

Great Meat Loaf
6 servings

This recipe produces a moist, delicious meat loaf. It makes six diet-size portions and leftovers can be refrigerated for later use.

Ingredients	Amount
Ground beef (70% / 30%)	1 lb.
Unflavored pork rinds	1 cup (about ¾ oz)
Large egg	1
Salt	to taste
Low-carb ketchup (Heinz™)	2 tablespoons
Mustard	1 teaspoon
Non-calorie brown sugar substitute (Sugar Twin™)	1 tablespoon, to taste

Instructions: Crush the pork rinds into crumbs and mix in a bowl with the meat, egg, and salt. After mixing thoroughly, place in a loaf pan. Combine brown sugar substitute, low carb ketchup and mustard and spread as a topping over the loaf. Bake about 45 to 50 minutes in a 350° F. oven (or until internal temperature is at least 150° F.). If preparing in a microwave instead, allow about 14 minutes on high before checking temperature.

Energy	230	calories
Fat	16	grams
Protein	18	grams
Carbohydrate	1½	grams

Latin-Spiced Salmon

Salmon is a food that many recommend eating once or twice a week. This is an easy recipe that brings out its natural flavor. One important ingredient is Tajin,® a powdered Mexican spice often used on fruit. It is MSG-free and contains chili peppers, dehydrated lime and salt. If you can not find it, experiment with similar ingredients. You should be pleased with the results.

Ingredients	Amount
Salmon fillet *(small portion)*	About 3 oz
Olive or sesame oil	1 teaspoon
Tajin™	1 teaspoon, to taste

Instructions: Place fish in baking dish. Brush top of salmon with oil. Sprinkle spice over oil. Place in an oven preheated to 375°F (or 325°F for a convection oven) and cook for 15 to 20 minutes. Check to see that the fish flakes easily with a fork when it appears done.
Alternatively, this may be cooked in a frying pan over medium heat. Use extra oil in the pan and turn once when halfway cooked.

Energy	179	calories
Fat	11	grams
Protein	20	grams
Carbohydrate	0	grams

Lemon-Cheese Encrusted Tilapia

Tilapia is a light fish that develops a taste based upon how it is cooked. Since it does not contain as much fish oil as a darker fish, frying it will help balance the proportion of fat to protein. Its flavor will change radically, depending upon how it is cooked. Since tilapia fillets are very thin, this is an excellent choice for a meal that can be quickly prepared.

Ingredients	Amount
Tilapia fillets	1 or 2, about 4 oz.
Grated parmesan cheese	1 tablespoon
Dried lemon peel	1 teaspoon
White pepper	½ teaspoon, to taste
Salt	small dash, to taste
Sesame or olive oil (or butter)	enough to cover pan

Instructions: Grind the dried lemon peel to a powder (using a clean coffee mill or a mortar and pestle) or substitute MSG-free lemon-pepper. Mix the cheese and dry ingredients in a loose bag. Rinse the tilapia fillets and pat on a paper towel so that they are still slightly damp. Coat the fillets completely by shaking them in the bag. Heat the oil to a medium-high temperature before adding the fish. Fry for about 3 to 4 minutes until the crust is brown and crispy on one side, then turn it over and fry it on the second side until done. Serve immediately.

Energy	232	**calories**
Fat	15	**grams**
Protein	23	**grams**
Carbohydrate	0	**grams**

Halibut with Mustard Sauce

This tasty dish goes very well with steamed asparagus. The dressing adds flavor and balances the fat to protein content.

Ingredients	*Amount*
Halibut	4 oz portion
Olive Oil	I – 2 tablespoons
Real Mayonnaise	2 tablespoons
Mustard (powder or prepared)	to taste

Instructions: Cook the halibut in oil in a frying pan or alternatively, broil the fish after brushing with oil. Mix mustard with mayonnaise and top before serving. You may want to vary this recipe by substituting the creamy curry sauce for the mustard topping.

Energy	**345**	**calories**
Fat	**25**	**grams**
Protein	**30**	**grams**
Carbohydrate	**0**	**grams**

Recipe Worksheet

Recipe for _____

Number of servings _____

Ingredient & Amount	F gm 9	P gm 4	C gm 4	calories
1				
2				
3				
4				
5				
6				
7				
8				
9				
10				
Totals per recipe add columns	grams	grams	grams	calories

Divide the above line by the number of servings in this recipe.

Amounts per Serving	grams	grams	grams	calories

Cooking instructions & comments:

This worksheet is for developing your own recipes or checking recipes you find elsewhere. As you list each ingredient and amount, fill in the grams for fat, protein, and carbohydrate. Total these amounts, then divide these results by the number of servings to determine the grams per serving.

18

Questions and Answers

This chapter provides additional information and answers questions that people have asked. It may help to clarify topics that you have questions about.

Q. This plan sounds interesting, but I do not want to give up baked goods. I love bread and cookies. Why can't I follow this diet and still have them?

A. Sorry, this plan will not work for you if you can not give up those items. The carbohydrate allowance is very low for a reason. The large amounts of carbohydrates found in bread and cookies will be converted to glucose and raise your blood sugar. That will send you back into the deadly dance you were doing before, requiring medication, which in turn causes your body to demand more sugar. Fortunately, by following the plan outlined in this book, you will find that the seemingly insatiable craving for these items will go away. In addition, by using special recipes in the forthcoming companion cookbook, you will find that there are ways to create delicious very-low carbohydrate substitutes. Stay within the carbohydrate limitation and you should see those cravings disappear.

Q. I worry that all this fat will be bad for me. I would like to try this plan but skip the salad dressing in favor of lower-fat products. I will stick to skim milk instead of cream and use other low-fat dairy products. Will that be okay?

A. No, it will not! The whole point of this plan is to find the right proportion of fat, protein and carbohydrate to keep your body at its best fat-burning state. and your glucose at normal levels. If you skip the olive oil on your salad, you lose the benefit of the extra amount of healthy fat. In addition, if you use a typical "low-fat" salad dressing, it is likely to be loaded with sugar and MSG. The same thing goes for the dairy products with the fat removed. They will have carbohydrate calories in place of fat.

If you are a person who has an intolerance for fat, that is a special case. Go back and re-read the sections where I discussed gallbladder disease. Talk to your doctor if there is any chance of gallbladder disease and use some of the special medium-chain triglyceride products that are designed to be digestible.

Q. If carbohydrates and MSG are so bad, why aren't the people of Asia getting diabetes or overweight?

A. They are now both getting fat and diabetic. A 2010 study in China showed that in cities, more than 9 percent of adults had type 2 diabetes. That is almost the same as in the United States. The governments of China, Japan, India, and Taiwan have now recognized that obesity and the diseases it causes are wreaking havoc among their people. This is in sharp contrast to our image of malnourished Asians . Rice is a staple in the Asian diet but when poverty intervenes, quantities are kept small. Now that these nations are better off economically, their people eat more. A recent study confirmed that obesity among Chinese women is directly related to how much rice they eat.

Q. *I try to follow a low-salt diet. Is this diet low-salt?*

A. First, I must ask you if you follow a low-salt diet because your doctor recommended it? If so, your actual restriction is on **sodium**, a component of **sodium** *chloride* or common table salt. If you are on a sodium-restricted diet, it may be because of heart disease, kidney disease, or high blood pressure. You can easily follow this diet. In recipes that call for salt, use the substitute you would ordinarily use, which contains *potassium chloride* instead of *sodium chloride*. Since this diet avoids mono**sodium** *glutamate (MSG)* and uses smaller portion sizes, it already contains less sodium than most diets..

However, most people do not need to follow a low-salt diet. If you were *not* started on a sodium restriction by your doctor, you could hurt yourself by restricting salt. A few decades ago government officials began telling everyone to restrict their salt intake. Some health care providers jumped on that bandwagon, mistakenly believing that the bureaucrats had a scientific basis for their recommendations. The medical community has finally recognized that there was no sound reason for salt restriction in healthy people. In fact, there can be some pretty important problems caused by unneeded salt restriction. These include the following:

•**Hypothyroidism.** More than eighty years ago, health authorities in the United States realized that in many parts of the country typical diets lacked sufficient amounts of iodine. Iodine is a nutrient necessary for your thyroid to work properly. Iodized salt was introduced across the country as a necessary public health measure to reduce the number of people suffering from hypothyroidism. When government bureaucrats started pushing salt restriction thirty years ago, they forgot about the iodine issue. Today, health authorities around the world are attempting to increase iodine intake in diets by introducing or increasing iodized salt in the everyday diet; yet, in the United States we have inadvertently caused some cases of hypothyroidism by doing just the opposite. *Hypothyroidism causes weight gain and depression, among other problems*.

•*Chronic fatigue syndrome.* Chronic fatigue syndrome has become a recognized medical problem in the last several decades. About a third of the people suffering from chronic fatigue syndrome may have a low total body load of sodium. Because most of our sodium is stored in our cells, a simple blood test is not enough to tell if you are low on sodium. Instead, special tests done on a tilt-table are needed. *People suffering from chronic fatigue syndrome should avoid a sodium-restricted diet.*

•*Heat intolerance.* Before air-conditioning was common, it was standard medical advice to prescribe increased amounts of salt for people working in hot environments. Salt-tablet dispensers were located next to water fountains in athletic departments, military bases and hot factory work settings. Today, when athletes face this same dilemma, they are given sports drinks, expensive concoctions designed to replace salt tablets with salts dissolved in water with added colorings and flavor. ***Most of these sports drinks are loaded with sugar.***

Q. *I have been told to take a calcium supplement. Is that okay?*

A. Yes, extra calcium is important, particularly if you may be at risk for osteoporosis. There are many calcium supplements on the market. There are differences in cost and differences in absorption. I usually recommend a supplement that balances calcium, magnesium and zinc in a single tablet. These three important minerals can be found together in readily available over-the-counter supplements. Some also include vitamin D, which is necessary for your body to properly use calcium. See the discussion on Vitamin D in the chapter on supplements.

Q. *What is a calorie?*

A. A calorie is actually a measure of heat-energy. A kilocalorie is the amount of heat it takes to raise 1 kg of water one degree centigrade. There are actually different types of calories. The one used in nutrition is the kilocalorie, but in common use, it is just called a "calorie". What we are actually measuring in diets is a nutritional calorie or the amount of energy that your body can use from a particular item of food.

Q. Everything in your diet is pure and natural except for artificial sweetener. I would prefer not to use anything artificial, can you help?

A. My reasoning for artificial sweetener is that it beats the alternative. Sugar, whether extracted from cane, beets, or corn, does more harm than any other substance in our foods. If you have spent a lifetime of acquiring a taste for it, it may be tough to give up. Therefore, artificial sweeteners are generally better than the use of sugar. However, questions have been raised about aspartame, in particular. Most people who have a reaction to aspartame already are avoiding it.

Fortunately, the chemistry of artificial sweeteners varies. That means that a problem with or sensitivity to one does not mean you are sensitive to all. Read the labels carefully. Some manufacturers have started to combine multiple sweeteners. Others have switched the chemical they use under a particular brand name. If you travel overseas, read labels. Often, the sweetener used under a particular brand name changes from one region to another.

The best choice is not to use any sweeteners and relearn natural taste without the added sugar-taste. That is something to strive for in your children but can be tougher for you. I suggest that, if you are sensitive or wish to avoid artificial sweeteners, you consider using the natural calorie-free sweetener called *Stevia*. This is an herb, which you can even grow in your own garden. It is widely used elsewhere in the world, and is just becoming known in the United States. Although it has been available in limited amounts in recent years, recent FDA approval means that it is now becoming widely available and may show up in newer diet products.

Q. Why do you emphasize liquid sweetener?

A. Almost all powdered sweeteners **are not totally sugar-free.** As absurd as this sounds, in the United States, the law allows these products to be labeled as "zero calorie", "sugar-free", and "no carbohydrate" when they actually contain small amounts of sugar. Look at a package of your favorite "non-calorie" sweetener. The first ingredient is usually *dextrose* (a form of sugar) or *maltodextrin* (a starch made from wheat, corn or rice). These are there as a "flowing agent", simply something that attaches to the sweetener so that it flows like table sugar.

These amounts are small, so if you are having coffee outside your home, using the available diet sweetener will have little consequence. However, heavy use will quickly add up. This is particularly true if you use any of the products in cooking that pour and measure like sugar. The labels are deceptive, since they often show zero for a single teaspoon, but might contain thirty grams of carbohydrate if you are using a cup.

Liquid sweeteners usually are simply dissolved in water. Since they do not need a flowing agent, they do not contain these hidden dangers.

Q. I am a vegetarian. Many of your recipes contain foods that I cannot eat. Is there a way for me to use this diet?

A. Yes, dietary limitations, whether for reasons that are medical, religious, ethical, or simply preference can all be accommodated. The important principle to remember is to try to use the 60-40-10 plan. Since there are different types of vegetarianism, there is no one answer. Some people, who call themselves vegetarians may avoid only certain types of meat, while others may avoid all forms of meat and fish, and still others avoid dairy and eggs as well. The more restrictions that you have, the more creative you must be to get your necessary nutrients. Do not forget to take your vitamin and fiber supplements. If you avoid all meats but do eat eggs or cheese, you are getting good sources of protein. If you also avoid dairy, you may need to utilize tofu as a source of protein. Be careful and avoid carbohydrates, which are often present in large amounts in the vegetarian diets. Getting your fat from healthy vegetable oils, especially olive, sesame and flaxseed should be easy. Additional vegetarian recipes may be found in our companion cookbook.

Avoid vegetable-based imitation meat substitutes, which are usually highly processed soybean products, loaded with unnatural flavors and appetite stimulants!

Q. I am a type 2 diabetic but my wife is not. She simply needs to lose weight. Can we both use this plan?

A. Yes, you can change your lifestyles together. Because the 60/40/10 while in the weight-loss phase is the same, you can do that phase together. She may wish to read *Dr. Cohen's New Hippocratic Diet Guide: How to Really Lose Weight and Beat the Obesity Epidemic*, which is somewhat shorter than this book. Because you are checking your glucose and being monitored by your physician, you may find that you are stricter with yourself, but you will both do well. Once either of you get to leveling off, you may be slightly different in your needs, but you will both understand each other's plan.

Q. Is there a way to focus on my big belly?

A. Belly fat is a special case. Your expanding waistline might have been an early tip-off of developing impaired glucose intolerance years before you were diagnosed with diabetes.

When you are dieting, you do not have precise control over which areas you will lose from and which you will not. Exercise is one way to help tone you up, and it may help in the shape department. Different parts of the body contain different types of fat and some of these have hormonal influences on our health. In turn, they themselves can be influenced by our hormone levels. Keeping your glucose under dietary control while also losing weight will prove helpful in losing that intra-abdominal bulge.

Recent research indicates that an over-the-counter supplement called DHEA *may* help reduce belly fat. This was discussed in the chapter on supplements. It is definitely not for everyone, so discuss it with your doctor first, if you think you might try it.

Q. Why do you always suggest talking to my physician?

A. For non-diabetic dieters, I am showing my prejudice as a physician. Many will diet on their own and do fine, but a few people may not. Dieting is a highly personal act. Many will fear being shamed by failure and be reluctant to announce that they are dieting, particularly if their physician has not been supportive in the past.

You, as a diabetic, must work with a physician if you have been taking medication to regulate your sugar. Avoid the temptation to make this a do-it-yourself project, if medication is involved. The person to give you individual medical advice is your physician, not a salesclerk selling nutrition or diet products. If you are now taking medication for diabetes, your need may be reduced or eliminated following this plan. Continuing to take unneeded medication under those conditions would be dangerous and quite possibly disastrous.

Do not be embarrassed about talking about the weight-loss aspect of this plan. Your physician has seen many patients who failed at dieting, so plan on success and your experience will help others. My experience has been that physicians feel helpless when they see their patients fail to lose weight. Your success can be eye-opening for your doctor. A significant number of my patients are health professionals. Because of bad weight-loss information, they had experienced the same past frustration as you have. If necessary, provide your doctor a copy of this book before your appointment. *Together, you can decide if you are suitable for this plan, develop a plan for reducing medication, set your weight-loss goal, and monitor your progress.*

Q. I am concerned about cholesterol. Can this diet upset my efforts to control my cholesterol?

A. Surprisingly, this diet is much more likely to improve your cholesterol picture. The public has been confused by the pharmaceutical industry advertising. Cholesterol is an important risk factor but the early cholesterol medications could only lower both good and bad cholesterol together. This led to a focus on total cholesterol, not because that was the most important indicator, but because it was the only thing that these drugs could appear to improve.

Importantly, the emphasis should be on lowering *"bad"* LDL cholesterol while raising *"good"* HDL cholesterol. If you are on a cholesterol-lowering drug, continue to be monitored by your physician. I generally check cholesterol levels before people began this diet and after they have been on it for several months. Most importantly, look for the ratio of LDL to HDL. That single measure is one of the best predictors of risk.

Q. *Is there anything else that you can advise regarding cholesterol?*

A. Eating fish, particularly dark flesh ocean-caught fish for their omega-3 fatty acids, will help improve your cholesterol picture. If you cannot eat fish, you may want to take fish oil capsules. Omega-3 fatty acids can also be found at high levels in flaxseed oil and purslane. Today, other food products with omega-3 fatty acids are on the market.

The vitamin niacin is another powerful way to improve your cholesterol picture. Many doctors advise their patients to take this vitamin; however, it has to be taken the correct way. Taken correctly, many experts feel that niacin is better than the cholesterol-lowering drugs. It can lower LDL cholesterol while raising HDL cholesterol at the same time. Talk to your doctor about this option.

When niacin is taken by people who have not been told how, they will experience an itching or burning sensation, and their skin may turn bright red. Although this is harmless and it only lasts a few minutes, it frightens many people who vow to never try this again. The way to avoid this is to take niacin properly. That information is discussed in the chapter on supplements. Re-read it and check with your doctor.

Chapter 18   *Questions and Answers*

Q. I started out great, my glucose reading were normal within days off medication and I lost thirty pounds in the first two months. Once I got used to the plan, it became second nature to me. I love the taste of real food. My sugar readings remain great and my last A1c was 5.9. The only problem is I seem to have stopped losing weight. Some weeks I might lose half a pound and other weeks I'll lose nothing. What is going on?

A. If you want to continue losing weight, you may be too comfortable. Since your glucose is now well controlled, you have succeeded in reversing your diabetes, but inadvertently slipped into a maintenance mode. If you are still a distance from your weight-loss goal, I have to ask whether you are still keeping your daily diary? Information from your diary will help you find the answer to this question. There are two likely issues here.

Because you dropped thirty pounds, it now takes less energy to go through your daily activities. That means that your weight loss will slow unless you are also increasing your activity level. You may need either to adjust your daily food intake downward or to compensate through an increased activity level. ***Your body burns less energy after you have lost weight. This is not a problem, it is natural and you should plan to adjust for it***.

It is common to be lax about writing in your diary. Most people start out keeping their daily diary. After becoming comfortable with the plan, many people slack off. They may stop measuring because they get used to doing the same thing again and again. The daily diary tells the story, but if it has not been completed, it is impossible to figure out. Go back to keeping your daily diary as meticulously as when you first began. Look at the numbers. Can you see where they may have crept upward? It is often a small item that you have become so comfortable with that you stopped measuring. That seemingly small change gradually creeps up and knocks you out of balance. It may be that the cream in your coffee makes the coffee taste so good you have it eight times a day. It could be that a half ounce of nuts has gradually grown to four ounces. If you have been measuring and recording faithfully, you can review your diary and the problem may jump out at you. If you have slacked off, go back to keeping your log and you should spot the problem in a few days. *Making the extra effort to keep using your daily log will save you from many problems.*

Q. Eating out has changed for me. Several times I went to restaurants that I used to frequent but felt ill after eating. What is happening?

A. There seem to be three different problems which dieters repeatedly associate with eating out. You may have experienced any or all of these.

First, there is portion size. Portions that used to be perfectly acceptable to you should now seem gargantuan. After you have been dieting, your body will begin to return to normal and not accept those oversize portions. Your memory of what you ate in the past may trick you, even when your body is sending you stop signals. Use the hint given earlier about asking for the takeout box *before* the meal begins. *When you get served that huge portion, put some of it away before you begin to eat.*

Second, there is the sugar issue. As a diabetic, make it a point of remembering to check your glucose after eating out. Non-diabetics following the plan sometimes report that if they eat a sugar-laden desert, their thinking gets fuzzy, they get a headache, and they feel hung-over the next day. Their brains have gotten used to working from fat energy and the sudden change to the high sugar level of the large dessert forces them out of ketosis and produces powerful chemical changes in their brains. If done suddenly, it can feel quite bad. Remember, **only in our modern world have people eaten such a large concentration of sugar on a routine basis.**

Third, there is the MSG factor. Some restaurants really douse their food in MSG. The classic "Chinese Restaurant Syndrome" was first described about forty years ago. Because you have been inundated with MSG everywhere, you may have previously built up a tolerance to some of its immediate reactions, such as the headache and dry mouth that many people experience. After you come completely off MSG for a few months, you may notice the peculiar taste and sensation when you run into it again, especially when it is present in high levels. **This can warn you which restaurants and foods to avoid in the future.**

Q. Since I started dieting, I have felt calm, clear-headed, and better able to focus. What is happening?

A. This is no surprise, for many people report this same pleasant reaction. It is likely due to changes in your brain chemistry associated with ketosis. There are many ancient observations about this phenomena. Whether it is prophets in the desert or a medieval treatment for the mentally troubled, fasting has long been associated with mental change. Almost a century ago, it was recognized that these changes were associated with ketosis.

Ongoing research is looking at exactly which neurotransmitters are boosted by ketosis. These changes can be similar to those from pills, but more natural and without the side-effects. There has also been recent research into how diets high in fish oil improve mental health. Such research shows the power of diet over our mental state and may lead to radical changes in how we treat or prevent certain problems.

Unfortunately, this type of research is funded in a puny way compared to the billions spent by the drug companies looking for new pills. It is common to see overweight people who have been put on anti-depressants. Although I believe that many such connections exist, more research needs to be done to pursue these questions and provide alternatives.

Imagine the billions the drug companies might lose if something as simple as dieting could help millions of people now taking anti-depressant medications!

Q. Since I started dieting, I have lost pounds at a steady rate but clothing sizes seemed to drop in big spurts. Is this normal?

A. Yes, this is the experience of many people. As you move toward your final goal, reward yourself occasionally with new, smaller clothing, but be aware that you may continue to go down in size. Save the lavish spending until you have stabilized at your goal. Do not forget to exercise and tone up. Without that extra weight dragging you down, your posture will change and your whole physique will improve. This will also improve how you carry your clothing.

Q. I have occasionally noticed that my mouth is dry and sometimes I have a metallic taste or a sweet smell on my breath. What does this mean?

A. This is a normal chemical result of ketosis. It often is not noticeable and diminishes with time. If it is bothersome, a sugar-free hard candy or stick of sugar-free gum is helpful.

Q. My muscles seem sore after a long bike ride or run. What is happening?

A. Lengthy strenuous exercise often produces lactic acid. Ketosis can also produce acid. Usually, your system compensates for this well, but the two together may require your system to adjust more. Try dissolving half a teaspoon of bicarbonate of soda (ordinary baking soda) in a glass of water before exercise. Drinking this may provide your system the extra buffer it needs.

Q. How does alcohol fit in this plan?

A. Chemically, alcohol is slightly different but for the purpose of this diet, treat it as if it were a carbohydrate. Treat a glass of wine as if it were a piece of bread. If you feel compelled to have some, perhaps to join a toast at a celebration or for a religious observance, such as communion, remember that quantity counts. A small taste will do you no harm, but a full drink can easily upset your progress on this diet.

Q. *There is a lot of illness going around this season. What should I do if I become ill?*

A. Use common sense and listen to your body. If you are ill, try to keep your sugar under control, but remember that your body may require more energy to fight off an illness or heal. Weight-loss is of secondary importance. Do what you need to do, eat what you need to eat, keeping your glucose in reasonable control, and focus on recovering from your illness. Know what medications you are given, some medications (such as prednisone) are notorious for disrupting control of glucose. If losing weight, you will be able to re-initiate your loss after you recover from your illness.

Q. *When can I expect to find trustworthy food in the marketplace?*

A. This will occur when enough consumers demand it. Today, product managers for food companies see no advantage in honest labeling and trustworthy food. Some have said to me that they do not care what they sell, so long as there is "a level playing field."

These manufacturers believe that if their competitors bend the truth, they must do the same to be competitive. Unlike the past, where many family-owned companies had the sort of integrity you might hope for, food processing companies are now cost-centers of multinational conglomerates. If they do not pull the same tricks as their competitors, they will lose market share and their managers may lose their jobs.

Without improving regulation to level the playing field, it is unlikely that the food companies will change their behavior. It is up to you, as a consumer, to demand better.

> **"The health of the people is really the foundation upon which all their happiness and all their powers as a state depend."**
>
> **Benjamin Disraeli**
> *Prime Minister of Great Britain, 1877*

Q. What do I do now?

A. Congratulations. At the beginning, I asked you to read the book before staring to follow this plan. You are now ready to begin. I would suggest starting out in the following order:

1. Read the book completely. √ *Done*
2. See your doctor to plan reducing medication.
3. Develop your weight-loss goal.
4. Go shopping for food and supplies and clear your home of the wrong items.
5. Start the initiation at a convenient time.
6. Monitor your glucose, your fat-burning, and your medication use. Keep in touch with your physician.
7. Begin eating according to plan.
8. When you achieve your loss goal, switch to a diabetes recovery plan for life.

Annotated Bibliography

This section is provided for those who wish further information on selected topics. It is arranged alphabetically, by topic. A few items are referenced more than once, where they contain important information related to multiple topic headings. There are varying types of references here, since information about the underlying forces that effect our health are as likely to be found in the financial reporting of the *Wall Street Journal,* as it is in the medical reporting of the *New England Journal of Medicine.*

Appetite Suppression Caused by Dietary Changes

- Klein S, et al. ***Carbohydrate restriction regulates the adaptive response to fasting,*** American Journal of Physiology, Vol. 262 (5 Pt 1) pp E631-6, 1992.
- Arafat A. ***Glucagon Suppression of ghrelin secretion is exerted at hypothalamus-pituitary level,*** Journal Clinical Endocrinology Metabolism, Vol. 91(9) pp 3525-33, 2006.
- Arumugam V, et al. ***A high-glycemic meal pattern elicited increased subjective appetite sensations in overweight and obese women,*** Appetite, Vol. 50(1-2) pp 215-22, March-May 2008.

Basis for this Diet: Development of Mathematical Model

This diet was developed using a mathematical model I developed as an extension to formulas for maintaining ketoses on a non-weight reduction diet. The original work on those was done in the 1920's and can be explained using the formula:

$$KR = \frac{K}{AK}$$

- Shaffer PA. ***The ketogenic-antiketogenic balance in man and its significance in diabetes,*** Journal of Biologic Chemistry pp 399-441, 1922.

Annotated Bibliography

Research done by Woodyatt provided a mathematical basis for using this nutritional knowledge clinically. This is expressed by:

$$KR = \frac{(0.9 * f) + (0.46 * p)}{C + (0.1 * f) + (0.58 * p)}$$

- Woodyatt RT. *Objects and method of diet adjustment in diabetes*, Archives of Internal Medicine, Vol. 28(2), pp 125-141, 1921.
- Talbot FB, Metcalf KM, Moriarity,ME. *A Clinical Study of Epileptic Children Treated by Ketogenic Diet*. Boston Medical & Surgical Journal (now the New England Journal of Medicine), pp 89-96, 1922.

Based upon that earlier work, I modified Woodyatt's mathematical model to take into account the differences between maintaining ketosis on a diet in which energy requirements are being met and one in which the goal weight-loss. Using that model, I derived the following formula:

$$TKR = \frac{(0.1 * <e - [4 * (p + c)]>) + (0.46 * p)}{c + (0.011 * <e - [4 * (p + c)]>) + (0.58 * p)}$$

where:
- TKR represents total ketogenic ratio
- e represents energy needs in kilocalories
- p represents dietary protein in grams
- c represents dietary carbohydrate in grams

and when:
- energy deficit is met exclusively by the utilization of stored fat

- Cohen IA. *A method for determining total ketogenic ratio (TKR) for evaluating the ketogenic property of a weight-reduction diets*, Medical Hypotheses, Vol. 73, pp 377-81, 2009.
- Cohen IA. *Development of a Modified Ketogenic Ratio for Weight-Reduction Dieting*, Prevention 2006-Annual Scientific Meeting of the American College of Preventive Medicine, Reno, 2006.
- Cohen IA. *A Model for Analyzing and Reversing Historic Dietary Trends Which Contributed to Obesity and Its*

Resultant Disease Burden, Indian Health Service Annual Research Conference, Albuquerque, 2006.

- Cohen IA. *The obesity epidemic, metabolic syndrome and adult-onset diabetes: Combining a modern perspective and ancient answers*, University of Kansas Medical Center, Internal Medicine Grand Rounds, Kansas City 2007.

- Cohen IA. *Using a computer model to evaluate weight-reduction strategies*, Kansas Public Health Association, Annual Conference, Topeka, 2006.

Belly Fat: Relationship to Disease

- Jansen I, et al. *Body mass index, waist circumference, and health risk: evidence in support of current National Institutes of Health guidelines*, Archives of Internal Medicine, Vol. 162(18) pp2074-9, 14 October 2002.

- Woo J, et al. *Is waist circumference a useful measure in predicting health outcomes in the elderly?* International Journal of Obesity and Related Metabolic Disorders, Vol. 26(10) pp1349-55, October 2002.

- Fujimoto WY, et al. *Body size and shape changes and the risk of diabetes in the diabetes prevention program.* Diabetes, Vol. 56(6) pp 1680-5, June 2007.

- Chen Y, et al. *Waist circumference is associated with pulmonary function in normal-weight, overweight, and obese subjects*, American Journal of Clinical Nutrition, Vol. 85(1) pp35-9, January 2007.

Cholesterol: improvement on diet

- Hays JH, et al. *Effect of a high saturated fat and no-starch diet on serum lipid subfractions in patients with documented atherosclerotic cardiovascular disease*, Mayo Clinic Proceedings, Vol. 78(11), pp 1331-6, November 2003.

- Singh IM, et al. *High-density lipoprotein as a therapeutic target*, Journal of the American Medical Association, Vol. 298(7) pp 786-798

Diabetes: Dietary Treatment

- Cantani A. *Le Diabète Sucré et son Traitement Diététique*,

Delahaye et Cie, Paris, 1876.

- Ebstein W. *Über Die Lebensweise der Zuckerkranken*, Verlag Von J.F. Bergmann, Weisbaden, 1892.

- Newburgh LH, Marsh PL. *The use of a high fat diet in the treatment of diabetes mellitus*, Archives of Internal Medicine, Vol. 26(6), pp 647-68, 1920.

- Woodyatt RT. *Objects and method of diet adjustment in diabetes*, Archives of Internal Medicine, Vol. 28(2), pp 125-141,1921.

- Shaffer PA. *The ketogenic-antiketogenic balance in man and its significance in diabetes*, Journal of Biologic Chemistry pp 399-441, 1922.

- Dall'Olio G. *Il diabete nell'Ottocento La cura del Cantani*, G It Diabetol Metab, Vol. 27, pp 146-153, 2007.

- Westman EC, et al. *The effect of a carbohydrate, ketogenic diet versus a low-glycemic index diet on glycemic control in type 2 diabetes mellitus*, Nutrition and Metabolism, Vol. 5(36), 2008.

Diabetes Epidemic: Ancient India

Indian physicians were able to describe an epidemic of obesity and diabetes and identify its cause as sugar consumption well over 1,500 years ago. Recent research has validated the ancient Indian descriptions of type 2 diabetes described.

- Suzarta, as cited by Woodyatt. *Disease of Metabolism* (chapter of *A Textbook of Medicine, Fifth Edition*, Cecil & Kennedy editors) 1941.

- Kar, et al. *Prognosis of Prameha on the basis of Insulin level*, Ancient Science of Life, Vol. 16(4), pp 277-83, April 1997

- Hardy, et al. *Ayurvedic Interventions for Diabetes Mellitus: A systematic review*, AHRQ Technology Assessment 41, U.S. Department of Health and Human Services, 2001.

Diabetes Epidemic: Modern Worldwide Spread

- Yang W, et al. *Prevalence of diabetes among men and women in China*, New England Journal of Medicine, Vol. 362 (12) pp 1090-1101, 2010.

Diabetes Recovery

Diabetes: More Medication Can Lead to Higher Death Rates

- Gerstein HC, et al. *Action to Control Cardiovascular Risk in Diabetes Study Group, Effects of intensive glucose lowering in type 2 diabetes*, New England Journal of Medicine, Vol. 358 (24) pp 2545-2559, 2008.

Exercise: and Age

- Centers for Disease Control. *Percentage of Adults Who Engaged in Any Leisure-Time Strengthening Activity, by Sex and Age Group — United States, 2005*, MMWR, Weekly, September 8, 2006, Vol. 55(35) p 968, U.S. Department of Health and Human Services, 8 September 2006.

Fasting: Reduction in Heart Disease

- McClure BS, et al. *Fasting may reduce the risk of coronary artery disease*, American Heart Association 2007 Scientific Sessions, 6 November 2007.

Fat: Appropriate Dietary Fat Mixtures Protect Against Obesity

- Wang H, et al. *Effects of dietary fat types on body fatness, leptin, and ARC leptin receptor, NPY, and AgRP mRNA expression* American Journal Physiology, Endocrinology, Metabolism, Vol. 282(6) pp E1352-9, June 2002.

Government: FDA, Inability to Track Food-Related Problems

- Center for Science in the Public Interest. *Emergency Regs Needed for Tracking Produce*,
- www.cspinet.org/new/200807031.html (accessed 15 August 2008)

Government: FDA, Responsiveness to Public versus Industry

- Whalen J, et al. *FDA scientist attacks Avandia safety*, Wall Steet Journal, p B4, June 11, 2010.
- Asamoah, AK, et al. *Transparency at the Food and Drug Administration*, New England Journal of Medicine, 10.1056/ NEJMp1005202, 2010.

Government: FDA, Under Industry Control

According to the Organic Consumers Organization, the government official who approved a Monsanto report that purported to show the safety of milk from cows treated with BGH was the same person who had written the report for Monsanto. She was reported to have been aided by other Monsanto ex-employees then working for the FDA.

- www.organicconsumers.org/monlink.cfm (accessed 15 August 2008)

Government: Function of the Surgeon General

- www.surgeongeneral.gov/aboutoffice.html (accessed 18 Aug 2008)

Government: Health Objectives, Promoting Low-Fat Foods

Before the government began to implement this strategy, one out of seven adult Americans were overweight. Since the government has "successfully" promoted low-fat foods, two out of three adults are now overweight.

- Public Health Service. *Promoting Health/Preventing Disease: Objectives for the Nation*, p 75, US Department of Health and Human Services, Washington, DC 1980.
- Cohen IA. *U.S. Health Objectives for 1990: A Maryland Evaluation*, Maryland Dept. of Health & Mental Hygiene, Baltimore, 1984.

Government: Public Health Erosion in the United States

- Rest KM, et al. *Politics and the Erosion of Federal Scientific Capacity: Restoring Scientific Integrity to Public Health Science* American Journal of Public Health, Vol. 97, pp 1939-44, November 2007.

Hemoglobin A1c levels and Increasing Risk

- Selvin E, et al. *Glycated hemoglobin, diabetes and cardiovascular risk in nondiabetic adults*, New England Journal of Medicine, Vol.362(9) pp 800-810, 2010.

Inuit (Eskimo) Diet and Health

Vilhjamur Stefansson was a famous Canadian arctic explorer who lived among the native people of the north and learned their ways. He documented their diet and health and became an advocate for greater knowledge about these practices and their health benefits.

- Stefansson V. *The Fat of the Land*, Macmillan, New York 1956.

Industry: Collaboration between Food Industry Scientists and Tobacco Industry Brain Chemistry Experts

- Callahan P, et al. *Where there's smoke, there might be food research, too*, Chicago Tribune, January 29, 2006 www.chicagotribune.com/bussiness/chi-0601290254jan29,0,1306987.story (accessed 30 Jan 2007)

- Manier J, et al, *The Oreo®, Obesity and Us - Craving the Cookie* Chicago Tribune, 21 August 2005

- www.chicagotribune.com/news/specials/chi-oreo-1,1,5587986,print.story (accessed 8 Aug 2006)

Industry: Disregard for Human Life

Philip Morris (now known as the Altria Group) which controlled Kraft, was concerned that the Czech Republic might restrict tobacco due to concerns about health care costs. Their way of dealing with it was to commission the consulting firm of Arthur D. Little to provide a study for the Czech government showing the "beneficial" impact of tobacco. In addition to the taxes collected by the government, they pointed out the immense savings in pension and health care costs because smokers die younger!

- www.americanlegacy.org/Czech/print_czech.html (accessed 1 Nov 2001)

Industry: Fraudulent Labeling

- Etter I, et al. *Tyson ordered to pull Antibiotic-Free Label by June 18* Wall Street Journal, p B9, 4 June 2008.

Industry: Immunity from MSG Lawsuits

The proposed settlement of the class-action MSG suit known as *Eugene Higgins versus Archer Daniels Midland Co.* dated March 20,

2006 was filed in the Second Judicial District Court of New Mexico. Although the suit was purportedly about MSG price-fixing, the proposed settlement included a "covenant not to sue," which covered any suit by consumers against the MSG producers for any reason related to MSG. The final settlement, fortunately, limited this prohibition to the price-fixing question.

- www.msgindirectsettlement.com (accessed 27 June 2006)

Industry: Influence Over the Scientific Community

- Campbell EG, et al *Institutional Academic-Industry Relationships*, Journal of the American Medical Association, Vol. 298 pp 1779-86, 17 October 2007.
- Rowe S, et al. *Funding food science and nutrition research: financial conflicts and scientific integrity*, Journal of Nutrition, Vol. 139 (6) pp 1051-3, 2009

Industry: Ingredient Substitution and Profitability

- Jargon J. *Food Makers Scrimp on Ingredients in an Effort to Fatten Their Profits*, Wall Street Journal, p A1, 23 August 2008.

Industry: "Pro-Consumer" Groups Front for Industry

American Farmers for the Advancement and Conservation of Technology claims to "to educate, equip and empower all participants in the food chain to understand the benefits of technology and encourage consumers to demand access to high-quality, affordable food with a minimal impact on the environment." They do not mention they were organized and funded by Monsanto, maker of both recombinant bovine growth hormone and genetically engineered seeds. These are products severely restricted outside of the United States by agricultural and health authorities.

- Martin A. *Fighting on a battlefield the size of a milk label*, New York Times, 9 March 2008.

Industry: Preventing Small Producers from Identifying Pure Products

- Martin A. *State revises hormone label for milk* New York Times, 18 January 2008.
- Hightower J. *Monsanto fighting 'hormone-free' milk labels*

Topeka Capital-Journal, 29 December 2007.

- Carson J. *Milk labeling measure debated* Topeka Capital-Journal, 15 April 2008.

Industry: Public Relations Campaigns

The high-fructose corn syrup producers are not sitting still for increasing consumer awareness. Instead, they have initiated a major advertising campaign to make consumers believe that they produce a healthy product.

- Vranica S. *High fructose corn syrup mixes it up*, Wall Street Journal, 23 June 2008.

Industry: Soft-drinks and Supposedly Healthy Fruit-drink Substitutes Both Increase Diabetes Risk

- Palmer JR. et al, *Sugar-sweetened beverages and incidence of type 2 diabetes mellitus in African American women*, Archives of Internal Medicine, Vol. 168(14) pp 1487-92, 2008

Industry: Soft-drink Company Payments to School Districts

- Warner M. *Lines are drawn for big suit over sodas*, New York Times, 7 December 2005.
- Chmelynski C. *Districts' vending machine contracts increasingly under fire*, School Board News, 12 August 2003.

Ketogenic Diets: Clinical Uses Other Than Weight Reduction

- Wilder RM. *The effects of ketonemia on the course of epilepsy*, Clinical Bulletin, Vol. 2, p 307 1921
- Wilder RM. et al, *Ketosis and the ketogenic diet: Their application to treatment of epilepsy and infections of the urinary tract*, International Clinics 1935 pp1-12, 1935
- Talbot FB. *Treatment of Epilepsy*, 1 edn. New York: Macmillan; 1930.
- Freeman JM, et al. *The ketogenic diet revisited* In: *Epilepsy Problem Solving in Clinical Practice* Edited by Schmidt D, Schacter SC. pp 315-324, Martin Dunitz, London, 2000.
- Neal EG, et al, T*he ketogenic diet for the treatment of childhood epilepsy: a randomised controlled trial*, Lancet Neurology, Vol. 7(6), pp 500-6, June 2008.

Ketogenic Diets: Weight Reduction, Ancient, Hippocratic

- Littré MPÉ. *Du rêgìme â suîvre pour pedre ou gagner de l'embonpoînt*, in: *Oeuvres Complètes D'Hippocrate, traduction nouvelle avec le texte Greg*, Vol. 6, pp 76-9, Chez J.B. Baillière, Paris, 1849.

Ketogenic Diets: Weight Reduction, Nineteenth Century

- Banting W. *Letter on Corpulence: Addressed to the Public*, Third Edition, Harrison, London,1864.
- Ebstein W. *Corpulence and It's Treatment on Physiological Principles*, New Edition, H. Grevel & Co.,London,1890 (originally published as *Die Fettleibigkeit (Korpulenz) und ihre Behandung*, Weisbaden, 1882).
- Cohen, IA. *Weight Loss Advice of the Late Nineteenth Century*, American Association for the History of Medicine, Annual Meeting Birmingham, 2005.
- Cohen, IA. *Nutritional Analysis of Popular Historical Weight-Reduction Diets, Annual Scientific Meeting of the North American Association for the Study of Obesity*, (Abstract Published in Obesity Research, Vol. 13, Page A138, Sept 2005), Vancouver, 2005.
- Cohen, IA. *Analysis of Historic Medical Knowledge Concerning Obesity and Diet*, Prevention 2006-Annual Scientific Meeting of the American College of Preventive Medicine, Reno, 2006.

Lifespan and Diet: Ancient

Herodotus, circa 440 BC, recounts a discussion between dignitaries of Ethiopia and Persia, where the Ethiopians criticize the Persian use of bread, stating they live many more years by avoiding it.

- Rawlinson G (translator). *The History of Herodotus, Book III*, http://classics.mit.edu/Herodotus/history.3.iii.html (accessed 18 Aug 2008

Hippocrates, circa 400 BC "Those who are naturally of a full habit die suddenly, more frequently than those who are slender"

- Coar T. *The Aphorisms of Hippocrates with a translation into Latin and English*, A.J. Valpy, London, 1822.

Lifespan and Diet: Modern

- Masoro EJ. *Dietary restriction-induced life extension: a broadly based biological phenomenon*, Biogerontology, Vol. 7 (3), pp153-5, June 2006.
- Yates LB, et al. *Exceptional Longevity in Men*, Archives of Internal Medicine, Vol. 168(3) pp284-290, 2008.

Liquid diets: Ineffectiveness

- Tieken SM, et al. *Effects of solid versus liquid meal-replacement products of similar energy content on hunger, satiety, and appetite-regulating hormones in older adults* Hormone Metabolism Research, Vol. 39(5) pp389-94, May 2007.

Low-Fat Dieting: Ineffectiveness

- Shai I, et al. *Weight loss with a low-carbohydrate, Mediterranean, or low-fat diet*, New England Journal of Medicine, Vol. 359(3) pp229, 17 July 2008.

Mental Health: Brain Changes and Diet

- Noh H, et al. *Increased nitric oxide caused by the ketogenic diet reduces the onset time of kainic acid-induced seizures in ICR mice*, Brain Research, Vol. 1075(1) pp 193-200, 2006.
- Stoll, AL. *The Omega-3 Connection*, Simon & Schuster, 2001
- Simontacchi C. *The Crazymakers: How the Food Industry is Destroying Our Brains and Harming Our Children*, Tarcher/ Putnam, 2000.

MSG: Hidden

- Anglesey DI. *Battling the MSG myth, A Survival Guide and Cookbook*, Front Porch, Richland, Washington, 2007, www.msgmyth.com (accessed 18 Aug 2008)
- *Umami Enhancers: Monosodium Glutamate, Glutamic Acid, Vegamite, Worcestershire Sauce...*, Books LLC, 2010.

MSG: Increased Appetite

- Hermanussen M, et al. *Obesity, voracity, and short stature: the impact of glutamate on the regulation of appetite*, European Journal of Clinical Nutrition, Vol. 60(1) pp 25-31, January 2006.

- Hermanussen M, Tresguerres JA. *Does high glutamate intake cause obesity?*, Journal of Pediatric Endocrinology and Metabolism, Vol. 16(7), pp 965-8, September 2003.

MSG: Toxicity and Health Problems

- Schwartz GR. *In Bad Taste: The MSG Syndrome*, Health Press, Santa Fe 1988.

- Blaylock RL. *Excitotoxins: The Taste that Kills*, Health Press, Santa Fe, 1994.

"Natural": misuse in food labeling

The best way to understand the misuse of the word "natural" is to read this FDA docket on the red dye made from crushed beetles labeled as a natural product.

- http://www.fda.gov/ohrms/dockets/98fr/E6-1104.htm   (accessed 18 Aug 2008)

Obesity Epidemic: Worldwide

Estimated direct and indirect costs of obesity in the United States were $123,000,000,000 in 2001, but this is not just a U.S. problem. Worldwide, the latest estimates of the World Health Organization and the International Obesity Task Force are that 1,700,000,000 people are currently overweight.

- Hossain P, et al. *Obesity and Diabetes in the Developing World – A Growing Challenge*, New England Journal of Medicine, Vol. 356 (3), pp 213-5, 18 January 2007.

- Caballero B. *A Nutrition Paradox—Underweight and Obesity in Developing Countries*, New England Journal of Medicine, Vol. 352 (15), pp 1514-6, 14 April 2005.

Pharmaceutical Industry: Profits and Public Relations

Industry launched public relations efforts to maintain five billion dollars in annual sales of two cholesterol lowering drugs which were found ineffective by cardiologists.

276

- Rubentsein S, et al. *Schering, Merck Defend Their Drugs as Stocks Suffer* Wall Street Journal, pp B1-2, 11 April 2008.

Pure Food and Drug Act of 1906; Reduced Addiction

Before 1906, many people, particularly women, were ill and addicted to over-the-counter patent medicines and tonics. These contained a variety of dangerous drugs, but often these were hidden or secret ingredients. The passage of a law that required manufacturers to label these products had a tremendous impact. Although these drugs were not restricted for another eight years, many people who previously had no idea what they had been consuming stopped once they realized it was their supposed medicine making them ill.

- http://wings.buffalo.edu/aru/preprohibition.htm (accessed 19 Aug 2008)

Salt: Benefits of Iodized

The World Health Organization is trying to get the non-industrialized and developing nations to set higher standards for iodized salt. Although industrialized nations have been iodizing salt for about eighty years, Switzerland recognized that reduced salt consumption was undoing this benefit. They recently increased the amount of iodine in table salt. They then studied the health of pregnant women and children and documented the benefits.

- World Health Organization. *Recommended Iodine Levels in Salt and Guidelines for Monitoring Their Adequacy and Effectiveness*, WHO/NUT/96.3, World Health Organization, Geneva, 1996.

- Zimmermann MB. *Increasing the iodine concentration in the Swiss iodized salt program markedly Improved iodine status in pregnant women and children: a 5-yr prospective national study*, American Journal of Clinical Nutrition, Vol. 82 (2), pp 388-92, August 2005.

Salt: Limiting Restrictions to Those With Medical Needs

- Alderman M. *Dietary Sodium and Cardiovascular Health in Hypertensive Patients: The Case Against Universal Sodium*

Restriction, Journal of the American Society of Nephrology, Vol. 15 (S), pp S47-50, 2004.

Salt: Restricting Intake versus Balancing Use

- Cook NR, et al. *Joint effects of sodium and potassium intake on subsequent cardiovascular disease*, Archives of Internal Medicine, Vol. 169 (1) pp 32-40, 2009.

Vitamin D and Health

- Autier P, et al. *Vitamin D Supplementation and total mortality*, Archive of Internal Medicine, Vol. 167 (16) pp 1730-1737, 2007.

Appendix A

The Ancient Hippocratic Diet

Many questionable ideas attributed to Hippocrates go back many years. The ancient physician Galen, a Greek doctor who was famous for the surgical techniques he developed working for the Roman army, is partially to blame. Galen lived several hundred years after Hippocrates, but to impress the Romans, he frequently used the authority of Hippocrates in his own writings. Galen wrote in Latin, which became the language of later scholars. For many years, European understanding of Hippocrates' knowledge was limited to what Galen had said.

The Renaissance brought about tremendous change. Ancient Greek medical knowledge had been preserved but was found mostly in the original Greek or in later Arabic texts. During the golden age of Spain, Jewish and Moslem scholars provided Latin translations of ancient Greek knowledge to the Christian scholars of Western Europe. This rediscovery of ancient knowledge became an important part of the European Renaissance.

In more recent times, scholars have continued this tradition. This Hippocratic information on weight loss is not available in brief English language translations. Instead, it was a French scholar, Emile Litré, who produced the most comprehensive and respected gathering of Hippocratic works in the mid-1800s.

This particular Hippocratic technique focuses on how to

lose or gain weight. Although not specific for diabetes, it deals with the underlying issue of the causes of weight gain that are common to developing type 2 diabetes.

This Hippocratic technique for weight loss or gain is found in Volume Six of the encyclopedic work of Litré, *Oeuvres Complètes d'Hippocrate* published in 1849.

Major points of this Hippocratic technique, followed by my interpretations of their relevance follow:

1. Dishes should be fatty and glistening from sesame oil.

This clearly suggests increasing the proportion of fat in the diet, but emphasizes use of a healthy oil.

2. The dieter should not eat bread.

This is a suggestion to significantly lower carbohydrate intake. Bread was a primary source of carbohydrates in ancient Greece. Sugar was not the major issue at that time, since concentrated sugar extracted from cane was limited to India at that point in history.

3. These changes will satisfy dieters so that they are able to eat less.

This clearly points out the reason for the suggested changes was appetite suppression. No specific issue is made of protein, so if the amount the dieter eats is reduced, there will be a reduction in protein intake, not the increase found in some modern low-carbohydrate diets.

4. Eat only one meal a day.

In ancient Greece, there was debate as to whether it was healthier to eat two or three meals each day. Therefore, I interpret this advice to mean; reduce the number of meals that you eat each day. This is consistent with reduced hunger while burning stored fat. Conversely, those who eat high carbohydrate meals must eat more frequently to deal with fluctuating sugar levels.

5. Work hard with younger people

Exercise while dieting makes sense. Recent research shows, no matter what age group, younger people always exercise more. Therefore, working with those who are younger than you is a way to increase from your baseline activity level.

6. Sleep on a hard bed and stroll around naked as much as you can.

This sounds unusual, and I did not include it in my recommendations for practical reasons. However, it makes perfect sense. Sleeping on a surface without bedding will usually chill you, as will walking around naked. Research has confirmed that you have a higher caloric energy need when you are a chilled. Although it makes sense, it is not very practical for most dieters.

7. **To gain weight, a person should do just the opposite of these recommendations**.

Doing the opposite of these ancient weight-loss recommendations means that Hippocrates' suggestions to *gain* weight match what the government has told people they must do to *lose* weight.

Is it any wonder that dieters are frustrated when they followed the government's advice? Those who follow the government plan to *lose* weight are doing the very things that Hippocrates prescribed to *gain* weight. **Hippocrates' ancient work accurately predicted today's epidemics of obesity and diabetes.**

Appendix B

For Health Professionals

Thank you for reading this book. This supplemental section contains my opinions and experiences that I feel may be helpful to other health professionals. A number of the overweight and diabetic people I have seen have themselves been health professionals, spouses of health professionals, or referrals from other practitioners. You, like many of them, may be frustrated by the increasing problems that your patients are facing due to the obesity epidemic. You are well aware that for many of those overweight patients who have not yet developed type 2 diabetes, it is only a matter of time. You are also caught in the dilemma of tight regulation of diabetic patients forestalling some consequences, yet greatly increasing the risks of others.

The recent revelations that the government-sponsored low-fat diet craze is ineffective were probably not a surprise to you. When that research was published, it seemed like the small child (in the Hans Christian Andersen tale) crying out that the emperor had no clothes. The ineffectiveness of that government-sponsored low-fat fad had been obvious to most of us for some time.

Whether you see patients in a primary care setting, a subspecialty setting or another capacity, you have the ability to help your patients on their road to recovery from the dual epidemics of obesity and type 2 diabetes. Whether you are a physician, a nurse, or a health-plan administrator this should be important to you. It may have frustrated you at a personal level. When we can be successful ourselves, it adds considerably to the value of the advice that we give our patients. If you understand the basis for this plan and believe in it yourself, you can be invaluable in assisting your patients both to lose weight and to control their diabetes.

The basis for the weight-loss phase of this diet is the maintenance of a steady state of ketosis. Although ketosis in dieting is not a new concept, this plan is based upon a mathematical model for weight-loss dieting I derived from much earlier and widely accepted non-weight-loss research of others.

Fasting has long been recognized as having the ability to suppress hunger. It has been almost a century since ketosis was recognized as bringing about powerful changes in the central nervous system. Pioneering work done in the 1920s demonstrated that the seizure suppression properties of a fasting state could be replicated by a diet in which proportions of food were carefully monitored. The formulas developed at that time were not intended for weight-reduction. In fact, they were intended to create a steady state of ketosis without inducing weight-loss.

My initial effort was to extend those experimentally derived formulas to encompass weight loss. This allowed me to derive an extended algorithm that was helpful in predicting which dietary mixtures could maintain a steady state of ketosis while producing weight loss. The next step was setting reasonable limits so that total dietary fat consumption was not excessive while protein consumption was adequate. This resulted in the highly effective weight-loss diet first published as *Dr. Cohen's New Hippocratic Diet™ Guide: How to Really Lose Weight and*

Diabetes Recovery

Beat the Obesity Epidemic.

I had been and still am cautious in allowing type 2 diabetics to begin that weight-loss regimen. If they are already on medication, the need to rapidly decrease or stop all diabetic medication is paramount. Not doing so would likely cause severe hypoglycemia. Therefore, I only accepted such diabetics when they met the following criteria:

1. They had previously been instructed by the physician or health practitioner prescribing their diabetic medication about when they were to hold those medications. If they claimed they had not been so instructed, they were referred back for such direction. It was explained to them that they absolutely were not to begin this plan if they were caught between differing instructions.

2. They were willing to use their home glucose meters consistently and record all readings in their food diaries. During the initiation phase of the plan, they agreed to keep me informed by phone of unusual readings. I required them to sign an agreement about monitoring to emphasize the importance of this step.

3. I attempted to judge their psychological and emotional stability before allowing them to begin. I looked for their ability to consistently comply with this plan. In some cases, this involved judging whether they were coping with family situations that triggered binge eating or involved relatives who seemingly were deliberately sabotaging their diabetes control.

The success of this program among many of those diabetics has been amazing. Although conventionally diabetics are admonished that weight-loss will improve their control, most diabetics see an improvement rapidly, long before there has been substantial weight-loss. For those who have been on medication many years, this is powerful motivation to continue to be compliant. Those patients who accept that this is a lifetime plan to return them to health are pleased that they have finally found lifestyle changes that are both effective and enjoyable.

At the time I first developed this diet, nothing similar in the modern literature was accessible through Medline. Although there continue to be reports and studies of low-carbohydrate diets both for weight-loss and improved diabetic control, they often are based upon hit-or-miss diets, such as the Atkins plan and similar ones, without any underlying nutritional theory.

Since Medline (at that time) included nothing published before the mid-1960s, I had to search earlier literature to find similar diet plans. Surprisingly, those earlier plans were well accepted and well-known in their time. These led me back to even earlier work, particularly the popular but unscientific weight-loss diet of William Banting (a British undertaker, not to be confused with the more famous scientist) and the highly scientific weight-loss diet of Wilhelm Ebstein, (a well-respected German physician) both in the late nineteenth century. Fortunately, contemporary quantitative nutritional analysis of their diets was available. That analysis provided sufficient data so that my algorithm could confirm that those diets were ketogenic. Ebstein's work provided the link back to Hippocrates, through the 1847 translation of Emile Litré. Although there was no quantitative nutritional analysis from the time of Hippocrates , a qualitative evaluation of the principles of that diet shows that it should be considered ketogenic and similar in its effect of producing weight-reduction.

Diabetes Recovery

Searching further for similar ideas about diabetes led to the influential nineteenth century work of Doctor Arnaldo Cantani of Italy and once again to Doctor Wilhelm Ebstein of Germany. Both had been proponents of dietary control of diabetes. Despite the 1922 breakthrough discovery of insulin by Doctors Fredrick Banting and Charles Best of Canada, dietary control of diabetes remained important for most of the twentieth century. For type 2 diabetics, it remained the first line of treatment, with insulin therapy used where dietary therapy alone failed.

Effective dietary therapy began to decline with the development and widespread use of oral medications later in the twentieth century. As the oral medications required increased amounts of food, particularly carbohydrates, as a buffer to prevent severe hypoglycemic episodes, typical dietary education for newly discovered diabetics has been less useful in preventing the need for medication.

Because of this focus on medication, a small but growing number of diabetics have turned their backs on dieticians and physicians. Some newly diagnosed diabetics who wish to attempt to use dietary control rather than medication have instead been turning to alternative non-medical sources for information, sometimes with good results and at other times falling victim to false claims about magical products.

The paradox is that medical advice for strict dietary control should be increasing. The availability of the hemoglobin A1c test as well as home monitoring devices for glucose are two powerful tools that allow the patient and the physician a clear picture of what works and what does not.

The dietary issue was worsened by institutionalized fat phobia. A combination of factors was involved in that. First, the widespread notion that dietary fat (of any type) was by itself responsible for cholesterol imbalance. Such conclusions, when drawn from epidemiologic studies in the presence of high dietary sugar, reflect a powerful epidemiologic selection bias. Studies of the consequences of fat consumption where dietary sugar is virtually unknown provide different results.

The federal government's mistaken acceptance of the premise that obesity is the direct result of eating fat exacerbated the problem. By setting low-fat dieting as a priority national objective in 1979, they effectively limited research that would show otherwise. Today, such mistaken emphasis continues to hamper treatment. Government grants for groups at the very highest risk of diabetes continue to push this agenda, even though both the patients and the professionals administering such programs often recognize their ineffectiveness.

Today, we are beginning to see a change from the thinking of the past several decades. Today, there are studies documenting the role of dietary fats in improving HDL cholesterol levels. The anti-fat hysteria is beginning to give way to a more balanced view of the role of macronutrients. Yet, after a quarter-century of bad dietary advice from the government and the media, many people are hanging on to the very behaviors that made them obese, believing that they are doing the right thing.

In this book, I attempt to instruct people in a method which has proven successful for many people previously unable to help themselves. Some were candidates for weight-loss surgery or had siblings who had undergone such surgery. Many have had their general health and their outlook on life improve tremendously. Many were able to reduce their need for medication for chronic conditions. I hope that you can be supportive of patients who wish to follow this plan. If followed, you may be surprised at their progress.

Not everyone will want to come to you for your advice and support. I have attempted throughout this book to emphasize to the reader that, if diabetic, they must work with their personal physician, yet some will be resistant to doing so.

Some of that reluctance may stem from their previous weight-loss attempts. Previous dieting failures make patients reluctant to announce to anyone that they intend to try again. You may have seen so many failures at weight-loss that you are skeptical that any can work and feel helpless in your inability to offer meaningful therapy. Yet, your patients can benefit tremendously from your advice and support. You can break down these barriers by keeping an open mind and letting your patients know that you support their effort to help themselves.

Consider your role as a health professional as both an advocate and a teacher to your patients. You are no more immune than the general population in regard to the related epidemics of people being overweight and diabetic. If you or your staff need to work on his or her own weight issues, this is not lost on your patients. Conversely, professionals who have successfully battled their own weight problems are examples and role models to their patients.

Combining your professional skills with support, empathy, and perhaps your personal experience will be an asset to your patients. Once you see that success is possible for those you may have given up on in the past, you may find yourself reaching out to more patients. Simple screening such as waist measurement and BMI can be handled effectively by staff. Effective weight-loss and weight-control can become primary prevention for those you see professionally.

Should a patient come to you asking for help and advice, I suggest starting with an evaluation. I have just a few absolutes about who this plan is appropriate for. Three of these, specific to diabetics, were mentioned earlier. In addition, I never recommend weight-loss dieting during pregnancy. I also caution against dieting in women who are considering becoming pregnant. Nutritional needs during the first trimester are too important to take a chance on.

This book originally was intended for adults, although the principles of this plan are adaptable to overweight teenagers, particularly when they are showing early markers of impaired glucose tolerance and insulin resistance. Central obesity or polycystic ovary disorder in teens should be red flags to anyone dealing with this age group. I am aware of patients who have had their teenage children follow their parents' path in food choices.

Those following this plan should be reasonably mature and emotionally stable. They should be willing to give up alcoholic beverages during the weight-loss phase. Although many have succeeded despite having an occasional drink for a special event, those who continued to use alcohol on a regular basis have had a more difficult time.

Patients who currently need monitoring of blood levels of medication should be watched more closely than others. Dietary changes will influence some of these. Those on multiple medications for hypertension also require monitoring. Rapid weight loss can result in a reduced need for medication. Such patients should be cautioned to contact you if they experience symptoms of orthostatic changes.

When you meet with diabetic patients considering starting this plan, be prepared to have them hold diabetic medication as soon as they initiate their diet. Have them report their progress to you or your staff in those first few days. They may have some glucose elevation as they deplete their stored glycogen, but this should revert to normal or near-normal as ketosis begins. Some who have required multiple medications for diabetes, might benefit from Metformin for mildly elevated glucose readings. Avoid insulin or insulin-inducing medications, as this will reduce ketosis.

If significantly increased glucose readings persist, their diabetes may have been significantly advanced and beyond the scope of dietary intervention. In this case, attempting to use this plan in its entirety will be fruitless and should be discontinued. However, even back on medication, they can still benefit from the avoidance of the diabetogenic foods described.

Most patients have been able to normalize their glucose readings and A1c results, using either no medication or greatly reduced medication. Stress to them not to be complacent and to continue testing. This is not a one-time treatment but a lifestyle change. It is important to coordinate this with other professionals involved, to prevent these patients from receiving conflicting advice.

Many patients report a reduction in chronic musculoskeletal problems after losing a significant amount of weight. Occasionally, a previously very heavy patient will develop problems due to muscle spasms after rapidly losing weight. This appears be musculoskeletal compensation for the effects of weight that is no longer present. This problem should be treated symptomatically, but it is better to prevent it with an exercise regimen that emphasizes range of motion. I often suggest Tai Chi to patients. An excellent Tai Chi program has been developed by the Arthritis Foundation and may be available in your area. Other good options are supervised aquatic exercise programs and yoga.

Try to use percentage of body fat rather than BMI in weight when establishing a weight-loss goal. DEXA is now considered the gold-standard for this, but lack of insurance coverage puts this beyond the reach of most patients. You may wish to estimate body fat yourself or train your staff to do so. Not all methods are accurate under all conditions, so I prefer to combine the use of skin-fold thickness and an electronic bio-impedance measure of body fat. Some measures require only a single measurement and little calculation while others require up to seven measurements with complex calculations. None of these measures can be said to be totally accurate for an entire population. Therefore, I suggest that you use the best method practical in your situation and treat the results as an approximation.

Once you have determined the patient's percentage of body fat, it is a simple calculation to determine lean body mass. Working backward from lean body mass, you can determine a hypothetical ideal weight, if the patient were to lose no muscle mass while dieting. More information on doing this may be available at www.HippocraticDiet.com. Be sure to take the patient's weight history into account and set a mutually agreeable goal.

I review the following lab tests before patients begin :
- CBC
- Chemistry panel (comprehensive)
- Lipid panel
- TSH (with reflex T4)
- C-Reactive protein
- Hemoglobin A1c

In the case of diabetics, you probably obtain many of these on a routine basis. An impressive number of overweight patients who had not been previously determined to be diabetic will have C-Reactive protein and A1c elevated. Such abnormal results can be reinforcing for the patient, if they are presented with a frank discussion of the metabolic syndrome and the assurance that they will likely return to normal with dieting and weight-loss.

In addition, I test for vitamin D deficiency in a substantial number of patients. When an overweight patient presents with a history of any type of autoimmune disorder, recurrent infections, or chronic musculoskeletal complaints ranging from myofascial pain syndrome to fibromyalgia, there is a high probability they will be vitamin D deficient and benefit from adequate supplementation.

I recommend a sugar-free fiber supplement and a multivitamin to anyone beginning this plan. Other supplements that may or may not be indicated are discussed at length in the chapter on supplements.

In addition to your initial guidance, some people will prefer to diet independently, but others will benefit from an ongoing support group. You may wish to start a professionally led support group within your own practice or simply make available facilities for a patient-led support groups. Referral to a non-commercial support group, such as Overeaters Anonymous or TOPS, may be helpful. Losing weight is often more than just a physical act. The learned helplessness resulting from unsuccessful dieting may be replaced by optimism as they regain control over this aspect of their lives. For some, the physical change is accompanied by changes in self-esteem and outlook on life. There is often a brightening of mood.

For a smaller number of patients, the brightening of mood exceeds what you would expect just from these psychological factors which accompany their weight-loss. The biochemical changes that accompany natural dieting may come into play. These patients may truly have been sugar-addicted. Although there are observations of the effect of fasting on mood going back to the ancients, there is little research in this area. The possibility that ketosis can accomplish this should not be ruled out. The same neurochemistry changes that are powerful enough to suppress seizure activity may also change mood.

For these few patients, I recommend that they approach maintenance very carefully. I suggest that they familiarize themselves with available information on the impact of diets in high omega-3 fatty acids and mental health. Another possibility for them may be maintaining ketosis on an Inuit-style diet, emphasizing healthy fat while monitoring serum lipids .

I try not to discuss the many other potential medical problems attributed to free-glutamate flavor-enhancers. Instead, I emphasize the positive aspect of removing these hidden diabetogenic diet-busters. Learning to look for real foods and to shop at farmers' markets can have a tremendous positive impact on your patients' healthy eating patterns.

In this section, I have shared with you my opinions and experiences. I believe that the obesity epidemic can be stopped and the diabetes epidemic slowed, even if it must be done one patient at a time. Further information, and data sources for much of what I have discussed in this book, are included in the annotated bibliography.

Appendix C

Tracking your Progress

Use the pages that follow in this appendix as a diary. It is very important that you record your food intake, your test readings and track your progress. These daily diary sheets allow you to do this easily.

If you write the numbers in from every recipe you follow and every food you eat, at the end of the day you will be able to easily determine how close you are to your 60/40/10 goal.

Some people prefer to note the 60, 40, and 10 at the top of their respective columns. They then subtract the food value for each item as the day goes on, so that at any time of the day they can see how much remains at a glance.

It is not necessary to record calories, but you may wish to do so. If you do, the numbers 9, 4, and 4 at the top of the gram columns are there as a reminder. Multiply fat grams by 9, protein grams by 4, and carbohydrate grams by 4 to determine calories.

On the same sheet, there is a results column to track your glucose readings, your ketosis tests, and your weight. If you fill these out regularly, you will be able to see how closely you are following the diet, what dishes or restaurants keep you in ketosis, and what eating patterns help you to lose weight. Remember to compare morning weights to each other, not to evening weights, which will differ. Use the time column to record the time of test readings and meals.

The next page offers an example of how one woman did it:

- She entered the date and day of dieting, for future reference.
- She started the day recording her weight and test results.
- After meals, she subtracted her grams from the 60/40/10 reminders at the top of the columns, so that she could see how much she had left to work with during the day.
- Her urine test for ketosis was large in the morning but slightly less during the active day, when her body was burning ketones as fast as it was supplying them.
- Her weight went up slightly during the day. This is normal and the following morning it should be less than this morning.
- At the end of the day, she totaled up 64/39/7, which is reasonably close to her goal of 60/40/10. She was curious about calories, but did not have to put in their individual values. At the end of the day, she used the numbers at the top of the columns (9/4/4) to multiply the grams and calculate her total calories.

Following the diary, are two graphs. The first is a daily graph to use in the first few weeks of dieting. The second is a weekly graph. Both of them allow you to quickly glance at your progress over time. The diagonal line marks the amount of loss you would have at two pounds each week.

As you watch your progress and your weight continues to fall, you will have a reminder of what you have done so far, and a tool to point out when you are dieting at your best.

Additional diaries are available at
www.HippocraticDiet.com

Diabetes Recovery

Date: July 1		This is day 38 of my diet.				
New Hippocratic Diet™ Daily Diary						
Time	**Food Item or Test or Weight**	**Test Results**	**FAT** grams 60 x9	**PROTEIN** grams 40 x4	**CARBS** grams 10 x4	calories (optional)
6:30	weight	237 1/2				
"	glucose	97				
"	ketosis	large				
7:15	Coffee + tbs. cream		5	-	-	
"	omelet		11 (44)	6 (36)	1 (9)	
9:15	glucose	108				
10:30	Coffee + tbs. cream		5	-	-	
12:45	Salad, blue cheese		6	2	4	
"	Cream soda		5 (28)	- (34)	- (5)	
2:45	glucose	109				
6 pm	ketosis	moderate				
"	weight	238				
6:30	3 oz salmon/oil		11	20	-	
"	4 Asparagus		-	1	2	
"	Curry sauce		11	-	-	
"	Iced tea		- (6)	- (13)	- (3)	
8:30	glucose	110				
9 pm	Munster cheese x2		10	12	-	
	Daily Totals add columns		64 (576) grams	39 (156) grams	7 (28) grams	780 calories
Special events and comments						

Felt great during the day, had a high energy level.
Had 2 slices of cheese as a snack at night.

Date:			This is day		of my diet.	
New Hippocratic Diet™ Daily Diary						
Time	Food Item or Test or Weight	Test Results	FAT grams 60 x9	PROTEIN grams 40 x4	CARBS grams 10 x4	calories (optional)
	Daily Totals add columns		grams	grams	grams	calories
Special events and comments						

Diabetes Recovery

Time	Food Item or **Test** or **Weight**	**Test Results**	FAT grams 60 x9	PROTEIN grams 40 x4	CARBS grams 10 x4	calories (optional)
	Date:		This is day	of my diet.		
	New Hippocratic Diet™ Daily Diary					
	Daily Totals add columns		grams	grams	grams	calories

Special events and comments

Date:			This is day	of my diet.		
New Hippocratic Diet™ Daily Diary						
Time	*Food Item* *or Test* *or Weight*	*Test Results*	*FAT* *grams* 60 x9	*PROTEIN* *grams* 40 x4	*CARBS* *grams* 10 x4	*calories* (optional)
Daily Totals add columns			grams	grams	grams	calories
Special events and comments						

Diabetes Recovery

Date:		This is day	of my diet.			
New Hippocratic Diet™ Daily Diary						
Time	**Food Item** or **Test** or **Weight**	**Test Results**	**FAT** grams 60 x9	**PROTEIN** grams 40 x4	**CARBS** grams 10 x4	calories (optional)
		Daily Totals add columns	grams	grams	grams	calories

Special events and comments

Date:			This is day		of my diet.	

New Hippocratic Diet™ Daily Diary

Time	Food Item or Test or Weight	Test Results	FAT grams 60 x9	PROTEIN grams 40 x4	CARBS grams 10 x4	calories (optional)
			Daily Totals add columns	grams	grams	grams	calories

Special events and comments

Diabetes Recovery

Date:			This is day		of my diet.	
New Hippocratic Diet™ Daily Diary						
Time	**Food Item** or **Test** or **Weight**	**Test Results**	**FAT** grams 60 x9	**PROTEIN** grams 40 x4	**CARBS** grams 10 x4	calories (optional)
		Daily Totals add columns	grams	grams	grams	calories

Special events and comments

Date:			This is day	of my diet.		
New Hippocratic Diet™ Daily Diary						
Time	**Food Item** or **Test** or **Weight**	**Test Results**	**FAT** grams 60 x9	**PROTEIN** grams 40 x4	**CARBS** grams 10 x4	calories (optional)
	Daily Totals add columns		grams	grams	grams	calories
Special events and comments						

304

Diabetes Recovery

Time	Food Item or Test or Weight	Test Results	FAT grams 60 x9	PROTEIN grams 40 x4	CARBS grams 10 x4	calories (optional)
Date:			**This is day**	**of my diet.**		
New Hippocratic Diet™ Daily Diary						
Daily Totals add columns			grams	grams	grams	calories

Special events and comments

Date:			This is day	of my diet.		

	New Hippocratic Diet™ Daily Diary					
Time	**Food Item** **or Test** **or Weight**	**Test** **Results**	**FAT** grams 60 x9	**PROTEIN** grams 40 x4	**CARBS** grams 10 x4	calories (optional)
		Daily Totals add columns	grams	grams	grams	calories

Special events and comments

Diabetes Recovery

Date:		This is day		of my diet.			
New Hippocratic Diet™ Daily Diary							
Time	**Food Item** or **Test** or **Weight**	**Test** **Results**	**FAT** grams 60 x9	**PROTEIN** grams 40 x4	**CARBS** grams 10 x4	calories (optional)	
	Daily Totals add columns		grams	grams	grams	calories	
Special events and comments							

Date:			This is day	of my diet.		
New Hippocratic Diet™ Daily Diary						
Time	**Food Item** or **Test** or **Weight**	**Test Results**	**FAT** grams 60 x9	**PROTEIN** grams 40 x4	**CARBS** grams 10 x4	calories (optional)
	Daily Totals add columns		grams	grams	grams	calories
Special events and comments						

Diabetes Recovery

Date:		This is day	of my diet.			

New Hippocratic Diet™ Daily Diary

Time	Food Item or *Test* or *Weight*	*Test* *Results*	FAT grams 60 x9	PROTEIN grams 40 x4	CARBS grams 10 x4	calories (optional)
	Daily Totals add columns		grams	grams	grams	calories

Special events and comments

Date:		This is day	of my diet.			
New Hippocratic Diet™ Daily Diary						
Time	**Food Item** **or Test** **or Weight**	**Test Results**	**FAT** *grams* 60 x9	**PROTEIN** *grams* 40 x4	**CARBS** *grams* 10 x4	*calories* (optional)
	Daily Totals add columns		*grams*	*grams*	*grams*	*calories*

Special events and comments

Diabetes Recovery

Date:			This is day		of my diet.	
New Hippocratic Diet™ Daily Diary						
Time	**Food Item** *or Test* *or Weight*	**Test** **Results**	**FAT** grams 60 x9	**PROTEIN** grams 40 x4	**CARBS** grams 10 x4	calories (optional)
	Daily Totals add columns		grams	grams	grams	calories

Special events and comments

Date:			This is day	of my diet.		
New Hippocratic Diet™ Daily Diary						
Time	**Food Item** or **Test** or **Weight**	**Test Results**	**FAT** grams 60 x9	**PROTEIN** grams 40 x4	**CARBS** grams 10 x4	calories (optional)
Daily Totals add columns			grams	grams	grams	calories

Special events and comments

Diabetes Recovery

Date:			This is day	of my diet.		

Time	Food Item or **Test** or **Weight**	**Test** **Results**	**FAT** grams 60 x9	**PROTEIN** grams 40 x4	**CARBS** grams 10 x4	calories (optional)
	Daily Totals add columns		grams	grams	grams	calories

Special events and comments

313

	Date:		This is day	of my diet.			
New Hippocratic Diet™ Daily Diary							
Time	**Food Item** or **Test** or **Weight**	**Test Results**	**FAT** grams 60 x9	**PROTEIN** grams 40 x4	**CARBS** grams 10 x4	calories (optional)	
	Daily Totals add columns		grams	grams	grams	calories	

Special events and comments

Diabetes Recovery

Date:			This is day	of my diet.			
New Hippocratic Diet™ Daily Diary							
Time	**Food Item** or **Test** or **Weight**	**Test** **Results**	**FAT** grams 60 x9	**PROTEIN** grams 40 x4	**CARBS** grams 10 x4	calories (optional)	
	Daily Totals add columns		grams	grams	grams	calories	
Special events and comments							

Date:			This is day		of my diet.	
New Hippocratic Diet™ Daily Diary						
Time	**Food Item** or **Test** or **Weight**	**Test Results**	**FAT** grams 60 x9	**PROTEIN** grams 40 x4	**CARBS** grams 10 x4	calories (optional)
	Daily Totals add columns		grams	grams	grams	calories
Special events and comments						

316

Diabetes Recovery

Short-Term Loss Chart

Day of Diet

Long-Term Loss Chart

Week of Diet

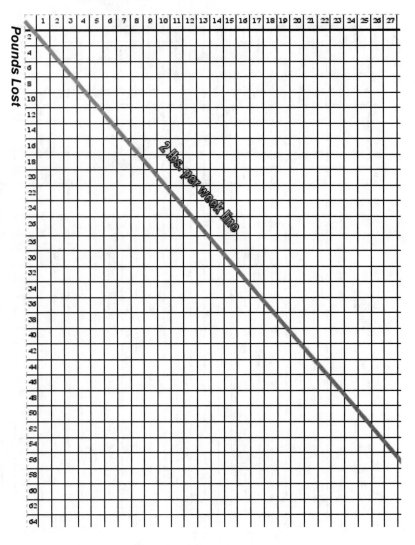

Index

A

A1c, 70, 72, 95, 176
  check periodically, 187
  test, what it shows, 47-48
Abdominal pain, 79
About the author, 342
Accepting success, 160-161
Acidosis, 88
Actigall™, *see Ursodiol*
Activity level
  continuance of, 176
  feel better about self, 168
  increase in, 170
  increase, and weight loss, 61
Add foods gradually, 174
Addiction Medicine, board certification in, 342
Addiction to high carb foods, 84
Addictive drugs, false triggering of brain pathways, 111
Additives, and food industry whitewashing, 214
Adults, plan for, 20
Advertising revenue, from drug companies, 46
African Americans, genetic curse, 4
Agricultural and chemical companies work together, 218
Alcohol
  and this diet, 262
  avoidance, 290
  beverages, clear out, 73, 101
Algorithm, for fat-burning state, 48, 266
All-you-can-eat restaurants, 150
Almonds, 145-146
  almond butter, 146

Alternative menus, 152
Alternative side dishes, 151
America, overweight in, 35
American Association for the History of Medicine, 19
American Board of Addiction Medicine, 342
American Board of Preventive Medicine, 19
American College of Preventive Medicine, 19, 342
American companies, sugar beet harvesting machine, 41
American Farmers for the Advancement and Conservation of Technology, 272
American Medical Association, recognition of Preventive Medicine, 26
American Revolution, sugar consumption, 174
Amish farm meat, and preservatives, 106
Amphetamine, as weight-loss prescription, 202
Amulets, and primary prevention, 27
Anchovies, fermented, 140
Ancient Greeks, and disease prevention, 25
Anemia from folic acid deficiency, 194
Annatto, 123, 143
Anorexia, 185
Antibiotic-free meats, 138
Anti-depressant
  medication, 186
  and overweight people, 261
Anti-hypertensive medication, 189-190
Anxiety, 83

Index

Appetite suppression caused by dietary change, 14, 265, 280-281

Appetizers, order, 153

Aquatic exercise program, 292

Arthritis,
caused by overweight,36
Arthritis Foundation, 292

Artificial foods, carbohydrates and flavor enhancers in, 37

Artificial sweeteners, 137, 174, 252

Asclepius, 25

Asian food and MSG, 107

Asians becoming overweight and diabetic, 248, 268, 276

Asklepios, 25

Asparagus, 133

Aspartame, 252

Aspirin and niacin, 199

Asthma, worsened by overweight, 36

Athletes, sports drinks, 251

Atkins plan, 286

Atkins, Dr. Robert, diet, 16-17

Author, information on, 342

Autoimmune disorder, and Vitamin D deficiency, 278, 293

Autolyzed
"anything," contains MSG, 123
plant protein, contains MSG, 123
yeast, contains MSG, 123

Avocados, 74
grilled recipe, 241

B

B12 deficiency, and folate deficiency, 194

Bacon, MSG-free, 74
rinds, unflavored, 146-147, 242

Bad messages, ignore, 168

Baked goods, 247
clear out, 73, 101

Baking cocoa, 74

Baking goods, and hydrogenated fats, 117

Baking soda, see Bicarbonate

Banting, Frederick, discovery of insulin, 42

Banting, William, diet author 286, 287

Barbecue sauce, 137, 232

Barley malt, 123

Balsamic vinegar, avoidance, 135

Bats, 107

Bathroom scale, 69, 75

Beans, avoiding, 73-74, 101, 134, 182

Beet sugar, cane sugar substitute, 120

Beets, skip, 134

Belly fat, 69, 255
relationship to disease, 267

Best, Charles, discovery of insulin, 42, 287

Beverages, 144
to clear out, 205

BGH, 210

Bibliothéque Interuniversitaire de Medécine, viii

Bicarbonate, added to diet, 60, 88, 262

Binge

Binge eating, 285
and this diet, 71
binge eating disorder, 49

Biochemical change from weight loss, 294

Bipolar disorder, and dieting, 23

Bleu cheese, 143
dip or dressing, 86, 154, 229

Blindness, and tertiary prevention, 30

Blood pressure
medication, 189-190
monitoring sitting and standing, 190

Blood sugar control,
and reversing diabetes, 1-2
less organ damage, 2

Blood sugar monitoring
after eating, 90-91
and additions to diet, 185
and diet, 59
close monitoring of, 170
measurement, 70
tracking, 176

BMI, see Body-mass index

Board certification of Dr. Cohen, 19

Body parts and different types of fat, 255

Body-fat measuring, 69

Index

Index

Index

Index

Index

Indian Health Service, U.S. Department of Interior, 19

Industry and professional organizations, ties between, 47

Industry, *see* Food industry

Infections recurrent, and Vitamin D deficiency, 293

Infections, and tertiary prevention, 30

Ingredient substitution, and food industry profits, 272

Ingredients,
list, by quantity of product in them, 126
list, shortest, 125, 126
out of place for food they are in, possibly contains MSG, 123
you do not understand, avoid, 125

Inositol hexaniotinate, 198

Insulin,
and fat storage, 6
and glucagon, 51-52
resistance, 14-15, 29
resistance, developing, 43
resistance, progressing to insulin insufficiency, 49-50
therapy, and needles, 42

Insulin-glucagon balance, 54

Internet advice, 10

Inuit diet, 186

Inuit diets, 271

Inuit-type diet, 294

Inulin fiber, 77

Iodine, 190, 200-20,
deficiency and hypothyroidism, 200
lack of in food, 249-250

Iodized salt, 250

Irritable bowel syndrome, 174, 182

Japan, obesity and disease in, 248

Jell-O™ *(sugar free), 74,*
for fat-centered partial fast, 86

Jesus and fasting, 55

Johns Hopkins University, 18-19, 342

Jolly fat lady stereotype, 160

Juice boxes, 205

Junk food, clear out of house, 204-205

K

Kansas clinics, 19

Karl Menninger School of Psychiatry and Mental Health, 342

Ketchup, 137

Ketogenic diets,
and Hippocrates, 274
and weight loss, 56
earlier, 286
going off and depression, 186
nineteenth century, 274

Ketogenic diets, uses other than weight loss, 186, 273-274

Ketogenic food mixtures, 19

Ketone test strips, 75, 77,
use of, 87-88

Ketosis,
and brain chemistry, 260-261
and emergencies, 60
and ketones in bloodstream, 56
and mellow feeling, 83
and mental state, 185
and well-being, 185
as normal condition, 60
basis of weight loss, 284
produces lactic acid, 262
signals fat burning and suppresses hunger, 56

Ketostix™, 77

Kidney disease, caused by overweight, 36

Kidney failure, and tertiary prevention, 30

Kilocalorie, 251

Kitchen diet scale, 75-76

Kombu, 107

Kosher meats, 139

Kraft™, 271

L

Lab tests before diet, 292

Labeling of food, 208

Labeling, fraudulent in food industry, 271

Labels, read all suspiciously, 100

M

Index

Index

Index

TOPS, 164, 182, 293

Tracking your progress, 295-305

Trade groups, front phony organizations, 10

Trans fat,
clear out, 73, 101
unhealthiest fats, 117, 118

Trigger foods, 171, 175, 182

Trips,
avoid being stupid, 157
enjoy, 157-158

Tropical oil, 118

Trustworthy food in the marketplace, 263-264

Tuberculosis, and Vitamin D, 192-193

Tuesday meal plan, 222

Tuna, *see also* Canned tuna,
canned, usually contains MSG, 116
canned, contains MSG, 116

Turkeys, 179

Type 1 diabetes, insulin for, 42

Type 1 diabetic, 82

Type 2 diabetes,
and genetics, 4
and insulin resistance, 14
and tertiary prevention, 30
known as Prameha, vii-viii
natural reversal of, 30
diets, 39

Type 2 diabetics
and ketosis, 88
and nondiabetics on this diet, 254
and fat burning state, 8-9
among doctor's patients, 283

U

U.S. Food and Drug Administration, *see* FDA

U.S. Government dietary guidelines, 176

Ultra-pasteurized "anything," 123

Ultra-pasteurized cream, 143

Umami, "tasty receptor," 110, 112

Unhealthy fats, 117

United States,
public health erosion in, 270
sugar consumption in, 43
type 2 diabetes in, 248

University of Kansas School of Medicine, 19, 342

Unsalted sweet butter, additives in, 143

Upset, and eating link, 49

Urine differences on fat-burning diet, 87

Urine testing

Urine testing,
for ketosis, 59-60
versus blood testing, 87

Ursodeoxycholic acid, *see* Ursodiol

Ursodiol, 78

USDA food pyramid, 183

V

"Vegetable broth," form of MSG, 114, 123

Vegetable oils,
and hydrogenated, 118
avoid generic, 135
replace more costly fats, 102-103
source of trans-fat, 118

"Vegetable protein," form of MSG, 114

Vegetable-based imitation meat substitutes, 254

Vegetables,
in maintenance diet, 182
shopping, 137-138

Vegetarians,
and carnitine deficiency, 197
and this diet, 253-254

Vinegars,
avoid balsamic, 135
shopping for, 135

Virgin olive oil, 74

Vitamin and mineral supplements (sugar free), on calorie-free fast, 85

Vitamin B-12 deficiency,
after stomach surgery, 196
in non-meat eaters, 196

Vitamin D, 192-193, 251,
amount needed, 193
and health, 278
blood test for , 193
bone growth, 192
D3, cholecalciferol, 193
deficiency, 293
regulating immune system, 192-193

Index

About the Author

Irving Cohen, M.D., M.P.H. is a physician who has dedicated his medical career to the prevention of disease, focusing on early detection and interventions to prevent later serious diseases. He directs Preventive Medicine Associates and serves as a volunteer physician serving the uninsured at the Marian Clinic of the Little Sisters of Charity. He and his wife, Lauren, have resided in Kansas almost twenty years.

Earlier, he had retired but became interested in the emerging epidemics of overweight and diabetes. His research prompted his return to practice.

Dr. Cohen has served in private practice and government service, in public health and clinical medicine. He has served as Deputy Director of the New York State Research Institute on Addiction. He held faculty appointments at the State University of New York at Buffalo, School of Medicine, in both the Departments of Medicine as well as Social and Preventive Medicine. He has held faculty appointments at the University of Kansas, School of Medicine in the Department of the History of Medicine as well as the Department of Preventive Medicine. He held a faculty appointment at the Karl Menninger School of Psychiatry and Mental Health Sciences.

Dr. Cohen received his training in Preventive Medicine and Public Health at the Johns Hopkins University, Bloomberg School of Public Health in Baltimore, Maryland. He served as Chief Resident of Preventive Medicine at that institution. Dr. Cohen is a Fellow of the American College of Preventive Medicine. He is Board-Certified in Preventive Medicine and Public Health by the American Board of Preventive Medicine and is also Board-Certified in Addiction Medicine by the American Board of Addiction Medicine.